START
YOUR
ENGINES

SAM BRIGGS

START YOUR ENGINES

EBURY
PRESS

1

Ebury Press, an imprint of Ebury Publishing
20 Vauxhall Bridge Road
London SW1V 2SA

Ebury Press is part of the Penguin Random House group of companies whose
addresses can be found at global.penguinrandomhouse.com

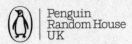

First published by Ebury Press in 2020
This paperback edition published in 2021

www.penguin.co.uk

A CIP catalogue record for this book is available from the British Library

ISBN 9781529105919

Typeset in 9.42/15.45 pt ITC Galliard Std
by Integra Software Services Pvt. Ltd, Pondicherry

Printed and bound in Italy by Grafica Veneta S.p.A.

The authorised representative in the EEA is Penguin Random House Ireland,
Morrison Chambers, 32 Nassau Street, Dublin D02 YH68.

For my mum for putting up with me and always encouraging me to follow my dreams

CONTENTS

INTRODUCTION: SPIRIT OF THE GAMES

Whenever the CrossFit Games come to an end, I always get a bit emotional. It's like the end of a really good holiday, except instead of going with your family or some friends there's a group of about 25,000 of you. It might sound a bit schmaltzy, I suppose, but that's exactly how it feels. CrossFit is all about community and this is our community's biggest holiday.

This year I was even more emotional as, unlike other years, something important happened right at the end. Not the podium bit. I didn't quite make it this year. No, this is something else that happens at the end of the CrossFit Games.

One of the most important elements of CrossFit is surprise. 'Okay, boys and girls,' they'll say. 'In one hour's time we'd like you to flip a huge tyre twenty times, swim 500 metres and then do fifty burpees over a giant hay bale while carrying a 70lb sandbag.' I've just made that event up, by the way, but I wouldn't bet against it happening one day.

And, boy, was I going to get a huge surprise when I attended the final ceremony this year. Every year the Spirit of the Games Award is given to somebody who has represented the sport well

1

normally over a number of years. It's the supporting act to the podium presentations really but, because it transcends just one event and is indicative of the sport, it tends to bring everyone together one last time. After that, the winners take to the podium and then we all go home, safe in the knowledge that regardless of how we fare in the coming year, either at the gym or in a competition, we'll always have, and be part of, our community.

The award is always announced by Nicole Carroll from CrossFit and, boy, does she have a way with words; she starts the announcement with a speech about the person who's going to receive it before revealing their name. Although it's easier to make a log cry than me, she always manages to make me well up a bit. As I said, though, this is the part that brings everyone together one last time, and as I was listening to her speech I realised it was starting to sound a lot like me. As she said my name, I couldn't believe it. Walking up to receive the award I knew that being a recipient would eclipse everything that's come before. Every win. Every PB. Every podium. It also reminded me of what we put ourselves through in order to be part of this community. The sacrifice. The dedication. It's all for the greater good.

When the award was announced and my name was read out, the wave of support I felt from the CrossFit community was overwhelming. The award itself is a mounted gold gymnastics ring, which, when I look at it now, reminds me of muscle-ups and, subsequently, all the hard work you have to put in to achieve the elusive muscle-up. Years of hard work! I'll treasure it. I'll treasure it forever. My favourite part of the night was Nicole's speech. I've never heard our sport described so succinctly before and once again she almost made me blub; it's a good job I'd already had a celebratory beer to calm me down! She reminded us that we as

CrossFitters have a common purpose of spreading health, whether it's creating the world's fittest or helping those who are facing challenges. She also highlighted the fact that physical performance is only one piece of the equation; what we do transcends aesthetics or points on a leader board and should inspire us, when we face our own challenges, to overcome them with courage, grace and resiliency.

Despite having one name on the front, this book, as with the Spirit of the Games Award, represents and is about an entire community. Our community.

I hope you enjoy it.

Sam Briggs, December 2019

CHAPTER 1:

A COMPETITIVE START

According to my mum, Karyn, I've been competitive from day one, as I arrived in the world three weeks early and before she'd even had time to decorate my bedroom. It obviously sounds like a joke but anybody who knows me will probably consider this to be true as I'm known for having an obsession with coming first. All I can say is, had I been aware that I was on my way into the world surrounded by others also arriving early, I'd have tried to make it four weeks.

Mum also says that I could speak, crawl and walk from a very early age and was inquisitive to the point where, if she left me unattended for more than a second, I'd be out of the starting blocks and off. I was into anything and everything, and if I got frustrated it generally wasn't because I was hungry, tired or grumpy. It was because there weren't enough hours in the day. Nothing's really changed in that respect and, if I didn't have to sleep to survive, I probably wouldn't. I've got far too much to do!

I was born on Sunday, 14 March 1982 in a place called Pudsey, which, if you're not from around these parts, is in the north of England. I arrived on Mother's Day and, because my handwriting was still a bit scruffy, my mum's best friend sorted out a card for me, which was kind of her. Pudsey is situated midway between

Leeds and Bradford city centres and has a population of about 22,000. When it comes to sportspeople, it's famous for producing cricketers, the most well known being Sir Len Hutton, who was captain of Yorkshire and England; Ray Illingworth, who was too; and Matthew Hoggard, who played for both and was a fast bowler. My grandad used to take me sometimes as he was a fanatic, but it wasn't for me. More crucially, playing cricket relies on a lot of hand/eye coordination and that's something I've always struggled with. Ask me to run somewhere or pick something up and I'll do it. Ask me to aim a ball at something or hit one with a bat and I'm afraid you'll be out of luck.

When I arrived on the scene, our family consisted of my mum, my dad, who is called John Paul but everyone calls him Paul, and a German Shepherd called Wolfie. My dad worked as a police officer and my mum was a nurse. When I was about one, we moved into my grandad and grandma's house on my mother's side. They were wanting to downsize and we wanted to upsize, so it was the perfect arrangement. Moving into that house is my earliest memory. It was a bungalow that had been extended upwards and I, shared later by my brother, had a room on the upper floor.

As a two-year-old, the only thing missing from my life, apart from more waking hours, were projects to complete and things to take charge of. So when my younger brother Paul arrived about two years after I did – again, this is according to my mum – I catered for his every need, whether he liked it or not. I moved him when he didn't need to be moved, I fed him when he'd already been fed and if anybody went to have a look at him in his pram while Mum was in the shops I would give them a potted verbal biography of his life so far.

'Hello. His name is Paul Briggs. He was born in April 1984 and he drinks milk, sleeps, cries a lot and poos his nappy. I'm his sister, Sam, and I look after him.'

It sounds sweet but I have a feeling it used to test my mum's patience occasionally. One day, when she was taking me to nursery, she spent ages getting us both ready and just before we were due to leave the doorbell rang so she went to answer it. She wasn't gone more than a few minutes but by the time she came back Paul was naked and back in his cot and I was standing over him going, 'You want to go to sleep, don't you, Paul? Off you go then.' Poor Mum went spare. It used to happen quite a lot, apparently. I wasn't bossy, as such. Well, perhaps just a bit. I think I was just interested in what was going on in life more than anything else, and I wanted to help.

While Paul was busy drinking milk and pooing his nappy, I was obviously on solids and my first spell in hospital, post-birth, was because I'd taken the 'solid' description a bit too literally and had eaten a Stickle Brick. I obviously don't remember anything about it, but Mum does. After seeing me put the Stickle Brick in my mouth, she tried to retrieve it using her fingers but unfortunately I'd already swallowed it. After rushing me to the local hospital, Mum told a nurse what had happened but there was nothing they could do. 'She seems fine to me,' said the nurse. 'When the Stickle Brick's ready to make an appearance again, it will.' I'm so glad I don't remember that happening as I have a feeling it might have hurt a bit.

A few years after moving into the converted bungalow, I asked Mum and Dad if I could have a room of my own. I was quite independent for my age, or so I thought, and surprisingly they said yes. I was allowed to choose my own wallpaper and my own bedding. Everything. It was brilliant. When I began moving my stuff from upstairs it started dawning on me that I was about to swap my cosy room, which I'd quite happily shared with my brother, for a new and slightly less cosy room all on my own. But it wasn't until I was sitting up in bed on the first night that the size of the new room hit me. I had a toy at the time, one that I used to love, and I was sitting there playing with it nervously. It was one of those toys that, when you pulled a cord, it lit up and played music, and until that night it had always either soothed me or amused me. Now, for some reason, it both looked and sounded scary and every time I pulled the cord I became more and more terrified. Why did I keep pulling it? I honestly couldn't tell you, but I did. Anyway, to cut a long story short, I lasted about half a night in my palatial new bedroom and, after I confessed to Mum that I actually hated it and wanted to be returned to my previous abode, she had the unenviable task of having to break the news to my brother. He'd obviously been thrilled to bits when I announced my independence and had been looking forward to my departure as any other brother would. Fortunately he took it quite well and we ended up sharing a room until we finally moved to a new house a few years later.

In addition to being intrepid and enthusiastic, I was also very sociable as a child, and because I liked taking charge of things and looking after people, other kids used to gravitate towards me. Not all, but the ones who were like-minded or were lacking a bit in confidence. That's something else I've never been short of, confidence, which is obviously the driver behind things like enthusiasm and sociability. From the age of about five I played for my local football team, and every Sunday morning prior to the match I'd have at least half the team in our kitchen for a pre-match meet. Mum would make them all bacon sandwiches and I'd get them drinks. Then, once I was happy that everyone had been fed and watered, I'd lead them all to the football field with our parents in tow. I played for both teams, by the way – girls and boys – and for the girls I played in goal and for the boys I played outfield. At that age you don't really have outfield positions as everyone tends to just run in the direction of the ball.

As well as playing football, I swam, played rugby, did karate and also tried my hands – and feet – at kickboxing and then boxing. I'd do anything, as long as it took some skill, effort and loads of energy, which I always had in abundance. If it was fiercely competitive too, all the better. I think my first ever sporting achievement was when I won my first swimming badge. They used to award them for distances and, every time I won one, I'd show it to Mum and ask her to sew it onto my Mickey and Minnie Mouse jumper. I still remember the excitement I felt when I realised I'd done enough to get a swimming badge. It was amazing.

The only thing I took up that didn't last during those early days was ballet. Unlike the fact of my arrival in the world three weeks early, anybody who knows me but doesn't know I did ballet will find it difficult to believe that it happened, but it did. Although not for very long. I think the reason I gave it a go was because Mum wanted me to try as many sports and activities as possible and so she enrolled me for just about everything. It was the same with Paul. I think I also tried tap dancing about the same time as ballet and, although I wasn't mad on the idea of either, a lot of my friends from school did them and that seemed good enough for me. It wasn't peer pressure, as such. I just wanted to see what all the fuss was about.

I went to ballet for a few terms and even progressed through a couple of basic levels. But I knew it wasn't for me and the instructor started to hint to Mum that I'd be better at other interests. Usually when I started a new sport or activity, Mum would be all enthusiastic about me continuing, and encourage me to persevere. Her reaction after my first ballet recital – the first time she'd actually seen me dance in public – was the polar opposite of this and the reason was pretty obvious. While everyone around me seemed to glide around the floor on a carpet of air, I sort of stomped a bit and made lots of noise. Grace and poise have never been my strong points, so it's fair to say that I was a bit out of place. I remember Mum walking towards me after the recital, or in my case, 'stompathon', and as opposed to looking excited like she usually did she looked horrified and a little bit embarrassed. 'You don't have to do ballet any more, Sam,' said Mum. 'Not if you don't want to.' Although Mum knew me, there must have been a little bit of doubt in her mind as to what my answer would be but, when I confirmed to her that I was extremely happy to ditch the tutu and ballet shoes, she breathed a huge sigh of relief and we left the hall very quickly. It should have been under a blanket!

To be fair, Mum should have seen this coming really, given the kind of sports I was normally drawn to. My brother went to the local Boy's Brigade next door to where the ballet lessons took place, so as soon as I had been released from the recital I happily joined him and ended up playing football with them outside. This was more like it! I obviously didn't get changed beforehand so, while the other girls were all being lifted into their parents' cars so as not to get dirty, I was chasing a ball around a car park wearing a leotard, a tutu and some ballet shoes. It was ace!

The person who usually bore the brunt of my flourishing competitive nature – in addition to all the girls and boys I played sport either with or against – was my already long-suffering brother, Paul. He was the one I always had to beat, although half the time he was probably oblivious to the fact. On the occasions that he found something he could beat me at, I'd berate myself for a while before letting it go and then I wouldn't play against him again. Learning how to let it go really wasn't easy as I obviously couldn't bear coming second at anything, so I would have to let him have his sports and I'd then go back to concentrating on things I could beat him at. In fact, forcing myself to move on when he did get one over on me was almost like an early form of sports psychology. Don't get me wrong, Paul was also quite competitive. He was just a bit more measured than I was and probably still is.

I think a bit of a leveller for me, certainly with regards to being competitive and always wanting to win, was learning how to play a musical instrument. Regardless of how talented or enthusiastic you are, you don't just pick up a violin or sit at a piano and start playing along to something by Tchaikovsky or Beethoven. That's why people often give up on musical instruments so quickly – they just don't have the patience. Fortunately, although I only took it so far, learning to play a musical instrument did help to temper my desire to want everything to happen immediately. It also helped to drive home the fact that if you want something good to happen – in this case it was getting a tune I'd been practising for weeks to a vaguely acceptable standard – you have to put the work in. It was invaluable really.

The first instrument Paul and I learned to play was the piano and I'd have been about seven years old. I remember our first teacher. He was really cool and quite young and, because he could play the piano really well, we were enthused and wanted to learn. Then, rather selfishly, he decided to move away, leaving us in the lurch. Paul and I were a bit upset by this, but Mum said she'd try to find somebody similar. She found somebody, but the similarities seemed to start and finish with the fact that they could both play the piano to a high standard. For one thing, instead of it being a young man who was quite cool, it was an old woman who was a bit frosty. Also, the house she lived in, which is where we had our lessons, always smelled of fish. So, after completing the short course of lessons Mum had booked, we thanked Mum very much and informed her that we wouldn't be continuing. To be fair to the old lady, the smell of fish was probably just her tea in the oven, but that didn't matter to us. It was horrid.

Our next piano teacher used to come to our house and because Mum didn't have to ferry us anywhere, and because we couldn't smell fish, the whole thing was a lot less stressful. This new teacher must have been at least seventy-five years old and, despite being really nice and good at what he did, he was also quite forgetful. This, I'm ashamed to say, is probably where I started to develop my skills in manipulation. The only piece I knew to any degree at the time was Beethoven's 'Für Elise', or at least the first couple of pages. At the end of the first lesson the teacher started talking about homework so I asked if we could learn Beethoven's 'Für Elise'. 'What a good idea,' said the teacher. 'Why not!' At the end of the next lesson, after we'd rushed through 'Für Elise' at the very beginning, the teacher started talking about homework.

'How about Beethoven's "Für Elise"?' I suggested.

'What a good idea,' said the teacher – again. 'Why not!'

This was definitely my mischievous side showing through as my brother would have just been happy to say he didn't want to do it. But between us we managed to get away with this for over three months. It wasn't the teacher who realised what was happening. It was Mum. 'I think we'll give the piano a rest for the time being,' she said. 'You can both try something else.' The reason I pulled the wool over my teacher's eyes was simple; I'd recently discovered the joys of playing out until all hours and wanted to be doing that, not learning the piano. It worked like a dream. Incidentally, I can still play the first two pages of Beethoven's 'Für Elise' with my eyes closed. I haven't practised for a while though. Not since I started having lessons at home.

The next instrument I learned to play was the cello, but it was supposed to be the violin. In music class at school you could choose an instrument to play and I'd chosen the violin. A friend of mine had also chosen it, which was partly why I wanted to learn it. So I turned up at home with one from school, took it out of the case, held it under my chin and, as I started making a noise that must have sounded like cats trying to sing a song while drunk, I told Mum that this was my chosen instrument. About two days later, my grandma turned up at the door with something that resembled a giant violin. 'This is for you, Sam,' she said, handing it to me. 'It's a cello.' I'm pretty sure Grandma was there when I brought the violin home and, because we spent so much time at her and Grandad's house, she probably thought, 'There's no way in the world I'm listening to her practise *that*!' All the cool kids played the violin, so when I turned up in music class carrying the damn cello everyone else just laughed. I was so embarrassed!

Because I didn't want to upset my grandma, I forced myself to learn the cello and I played it into high school. It did suffer one or two accidents, though. A bang here and a scratch there. I couldn't possibly say if these were intentional or not (on my part that is, not the cello's) but after a few years it mysteriously disappeared one day after being left, possibly intentionally, on a school bus. I think it was getting to a point where it was starting to interfere with sport and my social life, so it was time for somebody else to have a go.

As a general rule in my life, I am happy to push myself to the limits in those areas in which I have a chance of being the best, but I'm less interested when it's something for which I don't have a natural talent. Unfortunately, the cello joined ballet in that latter category – although you could also say that it heralded the start of my athletic career as carrying that thing was no joke!

CHAPTER 2:

JACK OF ALL TRADES

My biggest love in life – outside of playing sport and losing musical instruments – was always animals. For as long as I can remember I've always been besotted with them and it's something that's stayed with me my entire life. I don't think you ever stop being an animal lover. From the age of about four I used to find them and bring them home, something I definitely got from my grandma. The thing is, I would often find these animals before they'd actually been lost, if you see what I mean. It was a kind of fatal attraction for my four-year-old self. I'd see an animal, be it wild or domestic, and if it didn't have an owner within ten yards I'd attempt to retrieve it and take it home with me. Oh, look. There's a dog. I wonder who it belongs to? I can't see anybody. Here, boy!

The species or breed were immaterial. They just had to be not human. Cats, dogs, pigeons, hens – you name it, I used to give it a home, whether it wanted one or not. The ones I used to take the greatest amount of care with were injured wild animals and our garage used to be full of them. Mum used to cry, 'Not another one, Sam! What am I supposed to do with it?' That wasn't my problem. I was just the ambulance, so to speak.

To be fair, I did sometimes find lost or stray animals and the ones who genuinely didn't have owners would sometimes remain with us. I remember finding a stray kitten once just after passing my driving test. The poor little thing looked terrified and dishevelled so I took him straight home to Mum. We already had a cat and a dog at the time but I managed to persuade her to let him stay. Because he was in such a bad way, Mum didn't think he'd make the morning, but the following day when she came downstairs he was sitting on top of the curtain rail in the living room. He still lives with Mum, although he's not too good at the moment. Mind you, he is twenty, which in human years is about ninety-six. I'm dreading getting the telephone call.

Before I joined the football team and did karate, etc., I used to play all my sport and games on the street outside our house with the children from the neighbouring houses. I very rarely played indoors. There just wasn't enough space. There was a wall at the end of our garden and that would be used as a goal for either football or roller hockey. I used to love playing roller hockey. It was obviously different to football, in that you could pick up a bit of speed, and, although there were an awful lot of scraped knees and elbows, it was a great fun. If we ever got bored of playing roller hockey or football, which we did occasionally, we'd usually play something like Fox and Hounds. Fox and Hounds is like a mass game of Hide and Seek, but a bit more intense. It requires a large space to play it in and lots of players – preferably an even number. First, you divide the players into teams. One team will be foxes and the others are hounds. After that, if you haven't already done so, you set the boundaries of where the game can take place. In our case, when we were young we had to keep it quite local, but as we got older we'd spread it out as far as we could. Once the boundaries have been decided, the foxes are given a one-minute head start to go off to hide before the hounds go and find them. The game doesn't finish until all the foxes have been caught and sometimes it can go on for hours. That was definitely my favourite game.

The nursery that I went to fed into the local primary school, which meant that all the friends I made at nursery came with me. I don't remember much else about my very early childhood though, to be honest. Certainly not about my early years at primary school. It's all a bit of a blur and the reason for this is because I was always so busy. Kids tend to live in the moment so retaining information and making memories wasn't part of my agenda. According to Mum, I had no problem whatsoever leaving her at the school gate on my first day. In fact, I don't think I even looked back. One thing I did do, apparently, was come back out after the bell had gone to fetch my best friend, Hannah. She'd been the opposite to me, in that she hadn't wanted to let go of her mother's hand. According to my mum, who was standing with Hannah and her mum at the time, I came out, grabbed hold of Hannah's hand and pulled her in the direction of the school, saying, 'Come on, Hannah, you'll be fine!' Hannah was still inconsolable, the poor thing, but not for long. You never are in those situations.

But despite me running missions of mercy to distressed new starters and being ultra-confident with all my friends around me, I was about to have the wind knocked out of my sails. This I do remember! My new teacher looked the exact opposite to my mum and for some reason this alarmed me, big time. Mum had blonde hair and quite a deep complexion, whereas my teacher had jet-black hair and a very pale complexion. She also wore bright-red lipstick and I have a feeling that my fear of her might also have had something to do with me being a little bit suspicious of the evil Queen from *Snow White and the Seven Dwarfs*. Either way, my first year at primary school was all a bit much and I've probably blocked it from my mind. Funnily enough, I had the same teacher again about two years later and she was absolutely fantastic. I'd obviously got over my phobia by then and, rather than being suspicious of her, like I had been, I couldn't wait to get to school.

When it came to playtime I always preferred playing football and tag with the boys to playing hopscotch or skipping with the girls. Again, it just wasn't energetic or interesting enough for me and I had no problems at all infiltrating the boys' games. When I was young, Mum and Dad used to buy me dolls but, instead of giving them names and taking them out for walks and things like other girls, I'd cut off all their hair and then cover them in Biro tattoos. They should have just bought me an Action Man!

I remember Paul being given some Ninja Turtles for Christmas one year and I was incredibly jealous of him. My parents knew to get us the same things so neither of us was jealous but someone had obviously bought me something girly. 'But I don't want that,' I moaned. 'I want a Ninja Turtle!' To be fair, it didn't take people long to cotton on that I was a tomboy and at the end of the day I could always play with Paul's toys, whether he liked it or not. Mum says that she stopped buying me dresses from the age of about three. Grandma continued for a bit, but apparently when Mum tried to dress me in them I'd simply say, 'Not wearing that,' and walk off.

Despite being two years younger than me, Paul was always quite big for his age and, by the time I was four or five, he and I were the same size. He soon outgrew me, but until that happened Mum would save money by buying two-packs, so we'd be in the same jeans, T-shirts and even swim trunks. I didn't mind as long as I didn't have to wear a dress, but for a little while I'd be in tight-fitting clothes while my brother's would be dropping off him, which made for some interesting photos! I don't mind dressing up for an occasion, but I definitely feel more comfortable in jeans, rather than a dress. I'm also still a bit jealous of Paul as he went on to be over 6 foot, and for some reason I always wanted to be 6 foot. I've had to make do with 5 feet and 6 inches and I'm pretty sure I've stopped growing now. More's the pity. I also wanted to have really big feet though, I can't tell you why.

I also wanted tattoos. The reason I liked them so much was because art was my favourite subject and I was always quite good at it. When I found out that people could have things drawn on their skin with ink I was fascinated, and I have been ever since. They've got me into trouble once or twice, as you'll find out later, but even as a small child I couldn't wait to have one.

When it came to holidays, our favourite place was always the Greek islands. Grandma and Grandad had both worked in education – Grandma was a biology teacher and Grandad a chemistry lecturer – so they would have the long summer breaks and would visit the Greek islands for a few weeks. Because we were all so close it made sense for us to go as a family, although I'm sure it wasn't lost on my mum and dad that with my grandparents in tow they'd have ready-made babysitters on standby. Over the years we did Rhodes, Corfu, Crete, Kos ... I forget how many in all.

Pool time always played a big part in the proceedings (Mum and Dad needed a rest) but to let off a bit of energy we'd go down to the beach sometimes and have hole-digging competitions. From the grown-ups' point of view, it was a stroke of genius, as all they had to do was give me and Paul a spade each and then leave us to it! We would literally dig for hours. Incidentally, everybody says that athletically I'm an exact combination of my parents. Mum used to be a very keen cross-country runner, so I've got her legs, and Dad used to be a keen bodybuilder, so I've got his upper body. It's not a bad mix and it's served me well over the years.

As beautiful as the Greek islands were, my favourite holidays were the weeks we spent at Grandma and Grandad's house. They'd moved into a small house next door to a farm in Pudsey and on that farm were bikes, motorbikes, quad bikes, tractors, tractor lawnmowers, animals, hay barns and two boys who were about the same age as me and my brother. It was just a huge adventure playground and we had the run of the place.

Grandad and Grandma only had one spare bed so Grandma built a kind of nest in the corner of the room using duvets and cushions. A few years ago my brother and I were talking about this and all of a sudden it dawned on Paul that in all the years we stayed there it was always his turn to sleep in the nest and never mine. He was too young to realise what was happening, bless him.

The boys' parents, who owned the farm, employed a farm hand called Stewart and whenever we were in residence next door it was his job to look after us all. I'm surprised he stayed! To be fair, we always tried to help him as much as we could with whatever he was doing and in return he'd entertain us all and build tree houses. The only time things went pear-shaped was when it came to deciding whose go it was on the quad bike, which unfortunately was everybody's preferred mode of transport. One of us would always be left with a pushbike and whoever that was would spend all day playing catch-up. And whinging.

Sometimes the boys from next door would come to Grandma and Grandad's to watch a film with us. Grandma was usually the adult in charge and she would do arts and crafts with us but Grandad would often let us watch a film. One day this went horribly wrong as, instead of us choosing our usual Disney film, we selected one of his extensive collection of horror movies.

As I said, the boys from next door were about the same age as us so the older lad and I would have been about nine at the time and Paul and the younger boy would have been six or seven.

'What's this film, Grandad?' I asked.

'It's a film called *Salem's Lot*,' he said cheerfully, as if describing a light comedy. 'It's a little bit scary, though, so you might have to hide your eyes once or twice.'

Being so young, we had no idea what *Salem's Lot* was, but we were about to find out. Because Paul and I had been weaned on horror (Grandad used to read us horrors and ghost stories all the time), we were transfixed and just sat there munching sandwiches. The kids from next door obviously hadn't shared this upbringing and within about fifteen minutes the younger one literally ran from the house in floods of tears. The older one stayed but let's just say he didn't look happy.

'What's the matter?' asked Grandad, pressing the pause button on the video recorder.

'No idea,' I replied. 'I think he might have been a bit scared. Can we carry on watching it please?'

The boys didn't come back round for a few days after that. I can't think why! Needless to say, we weren't left in charge of choosing our own films from Grandad's collection again. He was absolutely horror-mad!

CHAPTER 3:

MOVING ON UP

The secondary school I went to, Pudsey Grangefield, was the same school my dad went to, and I was really looking forward to going when the time came for me to leave primary school. Unfortunately, my mum and dad split up during that first year of school, which was obviously a big shock. It's not something I choose to talk about normally, but at the end of the day these things happen, and you have to get on with life. My biggest concern after the split wasn't me or Paul; it was my mum. She was left to look after us both on her own and was also working long hours. Fortunately, she had Grandma and Grandad to help, not to mention some good friends, so all in all I think we coped really well. Mum certainly did.

One positive that came from the split was that it got us into karate. One of Mum's friends, who had two kids the same age as Paul and me, had also split up from her husband recently and, while on the lookout for something to keep us amused one day, they saw an advert for karate classes. As opposed to just the kids getting involved, the mums did too and we all had a great time. I ended up doing my purple belt but Mum, who took to it like a duck to water, got her black belt. Seriously, do not mess with my mother. She's as hard as nails.

I think Mum would have carried on practising karate had it not been for her job. She was now a bank manager (she'd started as a cashier while we were at primary school and had worked her way up) and after turning up to work with a black eye one day she decided that she might have to stop doing martial arts. She'd entered a competition the week before and, despite having to fight people younger than her, she'd got into the final. Unfortunately, her opponent was a bit more experienced and, although she gave her a run for her money, poor Mum had ended up getting a real shiner. Black eyes and broken limbs are frowned upon in the banking sector so that was it.

I'm glad she kept going for as long as she did because she ended up meeting her second husband at karate who's obviously now my stepdad, and they're still very happily married. I'm pretty sure I get a lot of my endeavour and determination from my mum as nothing really fazes her. When she went to become a cashier, which she did because we needed more money, she had no experience or qualifications in finance, but after working her way up to managerial status she was then employed as a crisis manager who had to turn around failing branches. She was like a banking ninja! I might be half and half physically, but when it comes to everything else that's needed to succeed in life I'm definitely my mother's daughter, and proudly so.

I'd pretty much outgrown my primary school by my final year there so I was excited to start at Pudsey Grangefield. The other reason I was looking forward to moving up to secondary school was obviously sport. Having already been to have a look around my new school, I was aware that the facilities were a hundred times better and so it ticked every box.

Despite being a sporty child, I couldn't actually categorise myself as one, if that makes sense. Not exclusively. The reason for this is that I was just as keen on the academic side of school as I was the sporting side – I think my competitive streak meant I just liked trying to be the best at everything. Usually kids were either sporty or nerdy, rarely both, and so in that respect I was a bit of an anomaly. Not that it mattered. I loved being interested in both sides as it meant my days were always busy and that was exactly how I liked it. It sounds a bit daft but if I could have covered everything at school – every subject, every sport and every club – I would have. I didn't just want to do everything, I wanted to learn everything. My favourite subjects were maths and science, and with those two subjects alone there was obviously enough to keep me interested. The more I learned, the more I wanted to learn. I was like a hyperactive sponge!

My first form teacher, Mr Curry, was a bit like my first piano teacher, in that he was cool and really laid back. He was also our PE teacher, so I used to get on really well with him. My other favourite subject was woodwork and that's the only class I used to ask if I could stay behind in. I didn't need to be given detention! I was in the top set for every subject at school but I would get the most satisfaction from something I would have to design and make. I remember making a pear once on a lathe and when it was finished I felt such a sense of achievement. I bet Mum's still got it somewhere – she'd better have; I was so proud of that pear!

The first thing I did on my first day at secondary school, after joining all the girls' sports teams, was to attempt to join the boys' rugby team. I'd played on the boys' football and rugby teams at primary school and for my local clubs, so I didn't think there'd be a problem. If you were good enough, it didn't matter, right?

How wrong was I? The teacher in charge immediately put me in my place when I told him I wanted to join.

'Girls aren't allowed to play on the boys' team,' he said firmly.

'But why?' I asked. 'There isn't a girls' rugby team in Year 7 so what am I supposed to do? I love playing rugby. I'm quite good too.'

'Be that as it may,' replied the teacher. 'I'm afraid the answer's still no.'

I honestly couldn't believe it. I don't think I'd ever experienced outrage before, not to this extent, but I was absolutely fuming. The closest I'd come so far to being outraged was probably after being sent to bed or something. In the end I decided to form my own rugby team at school and, although we were never officially recognised as a team, we used to train together regularly. If we ever got a chance to play a match, however makeshift, we did.

Luckily, my home-grown team was only a temporary arrangement as from Year 8 onwards the girls had their own established rugby team. The year of training on our own hadn't been wasted though, as we had really developed and improved in that time. Because we played rugby to such a high standard we were accepted into the same tournament as cub teams such as the Bradford Bulls and the Sheffield Eagles. The point being that these teams were coached by professionals and had everything that went with being associated with a professional team – the kit and the setup, etc. By rights a school team like ours shouldn't really have been in that league but as far as the bosses were concerned if you were good enough – and we *were* good enough – you were allowed in.

The reason we were so good is because we were basically a team of capable rugby fanatics as opposed to a bunch of girls who just happened to play rugby. One of our players came from a family that absolutely lived and breathed rugby league – from memory she had three brothers and a dad who played regularly and to a very high standard. They weren't going to let her be average, were they? Like me, she had also played on the boys' team up until the age when she wasn't allowed. As well as being fast, she had talent to burn.

Like so many good sporting teams we had a secret weapon. In fact, we had two secret weapons. I wish I could remember their names (I'm absolutely rubbish at names, in case you haven't already noticed) but these two girls were a rarity as they were very tall, very broad and were both mad about rugby. To have just one player like that in a girls' team is a luxury as they can change a game single-handedly. Having two then is just amazing and, because their enthusiasm for rugby was more than matched by their ability, we were basically able to take teams apart.

The only thing we didn't have that the other teams had was kit so we had to use hand-me-downs from the boys' teams in the end. These weren't the modern shirts that are made from polyester mesh. We had the old-fashioned cotton ones that looked like something from the 1950s. They were all far too big for us and I think this lulled the opposition into a false sense of security. At least at first. We would turn up looking like a walking history lesson and they thought we'd be a pushover, and of course we were anything but. We ended up finishing second in one tournament behind the Bradford Bulls.

The highlight of the season was playing a match at Odsal Top which for eighty-five years was the home of the Bradford Bulls. I read somewhere that the record attendance for Odsal Top was over 100,000! From memory we didn't have *quite* as many spectators as that there, but it was a fantastic day out and was, I suppose, my first real insight into how a professional sport works. I think we were part of the warm-up match for a men's first-team fixture, and all my family were there as well as a few friends. It was a big thing.

Rugby wasn't the only team sport that was vying for my attention in my teenage years. The activity that started taking up more of my life than any other at secondary school was football. I played on five-a-side and eleven-a-side teams and, between them, I covered almost every position except goalkeeper. In five-a-side I played defence or attack and in eleven-a-side I always played midfield. I had no preferences, though. I just loved playing and being involved. It was all a far cry from the early days when every outfield player, and sometimes goalkeeper, would just run in the direction of the ball. Finding out there were different positions and techniques involved in football was a revelation. You mean you don't just have to chase a ball and occasionally fall over? Wow!

In fact, it became my favourite sport and I started playing football for Bradford City as a schoolgirl. I think I was about fourteen or fifteen when I played my first match. I was invited to train with them one day, as were many people, and if you were good enough you got picked. Apparently I was and so that was it. I played a few games for them but my major stint with them didn't come until I was older and played for their open age team, when I spent a good few seasons with them.

At this stage, I still couldn't have told you what my future would hold, whether it would be doing something academic or playing sport for a living. Like most teenagers I was just open to everything and knew that whatever I did I would give it my all. Even if that sometimes got me into a bit of trouble ...

CHAPTER 4:

PUSHING THE BOUNDARIES

Anyone who knows even a little about my CrossFit career will be aware that I have been somewhat plagued by injuries. Indeed, this book is full of them. The first one I really remember happened in the sports hall during a PE lesson at secondary school in my first year. I think we were waiting for the lesson to begin and the teacher had been delayed so we were to warm up ourselves. To pass the time, we started playing football using the basketball and as we were doing this a friend of mine barged me into a wall by mistake and broke my arm. I didn't know that I'd broken it at the time, but it was pretty painful.

When the teacher arrived, I told her what had happened but she was mad we'd been messing around instead of warming up so she told me to stop whining and get on with it. It was already pretty swollen and bruised by this point, but I did as I was told and got on with the lesson – with a badly broken arm.

By the time the lesson had finished, my arm was about twice its normal size and with the pain now increasing by the minute she sent me to go and see the school nurse. Fortunately, she could see my predicament and, after she put my arm in ice and rang my grandma (who had a car), I was taken to hospital. To be fair to the teacher, she did apologise afterwards for not taking me seriously. It was just one of those things. She did actually start a trend though, as I seem to have made an art of competing with broken limbs.

Something else secondary school introduced me to, apart from wooden pears and broken limbs, was cross-country and long-distance running. I always preferred the look of sprinting when I was little, but I was never any good at it. It was the same with events like high jump and long jump. In fact, the shorter the race or event, the worse I seemed to be and again nothing's changed in that respect. Therefore, when it came to school sports days, I was always put down for the 800 metres and the cross-country, which was fine by me. As always, I just wanted to be involved and the longer I was out there the better. Had CrossFit been around in the early to mid-1990s and been accessible to people my age, it would definitely have caught my eye as my aim was always to try my hand at as many sports, events and disciplines as was humanly possible. I didn't have to be a master of all. Just some! The same applies to my early adulthood, as I was only introduced to CrossFit aged twenty-seven. But that's for later.

Mum always says that, although I was quite bright as a child, I was never very studious and that's probably correct. It's not that I didn't enjoy studying. I did. I just preferred exercising my limbs and muscles to exercising my brain cells. That said, I did put a fair amount of work in and because I had some natural aptitude I continued to do well academically, and I remained in the top groups throughout my school career. I'm sometimes asked if I had any aspirations to become a professional sportsperson while I was at school but to be honest I didn't. Once again, I was just too busy enjoying life to think about what I was going to do in the future. All that boring stuff was for grown-ups.

One thing that hadn't changed from my primary school days was my social life. In fact, if anything it had got busier, if that were possible. Once again, sport was usually the catalyst for these friendships and I'm still in touch with quite a few of these former team-mates today. In fact, five of us from school are meeting up in a couple of weeks for a reunion. Not all of us carried on being sporty. In fact, when we left school, just me and Vicki Wood continued playing football (we both played well into our twenties) but Haley, Toni and Gemma would come and watch us on a Sunday morning. That's real friendship! One of my school friends also came out to watch me compete at the 2011 CrossFit Games and a few have been out to the Regionals too. I might not hear from them for a year or so and then suddenly I'll receive a text saying, 'We've just seen you on TV!' I love the fact that they still keep an eye out for me, although none of them has taken up CrossFit yet. That's something I need to work on.

One of the few times I ever stopped talking as a child, and one of the few times I got properly told off by my mum, was when I had my tongue pierced. I was fifteen or sixteen years old at the time and, as soon as I'd had it done, I remember thinking, *Mmmmm, maybe that wasn't a good idea*. When I got back home, Mum wasn't in, so I just sat there and awaited my fate. One thing I hadn't bargained for was how tongue-piercing changes speech, at least when you first have it done. This was what alarmed me the most. So when Mum arrived home and started chatting away as usual, I just ignored her.

'What's up with you?' she said, looking suspicious. 'You haven't been drinking, have you?'

I shook my head while trying to look indignant.

'Are you sure?'

'Yeth,' I said with my head turned away. Or tried to say. 'I'm thure.'

31

Mum was onto me as quick as a flash.

'What's in your mouth?' she said, charging over and ordering me to open wide. 'Oh my God, you've had your tongue pierced! What is it? It's not a stud.'

'It'th a dithe, Mum.'

'A what?'

'A dithe!' I repeated, before sticking out my tongue.

'Oh, you mean a DICE! I can see it now. I don't like it, Sam.'

The truth is, neither did I.

I think what upset Mum was that previously we'd always discussed things and if I ever wanted to do something that I thought might have been deemed controversial I'd run it by her first. In hindsight I was just being a teenager, as most teenagers tend to rebel. On the other hand, I think I knew what Mum would say, so by not telling her I was just getting my own way. Perhaps they're the same thing.

Something similar happened when I had my first tattoo. I can't remember how old I was exactly, but I was in my teens and just like the tongue-piercing I got one done without running it by Mum first. Because the tattoo was small and out of sight she didn't go as mad as I thought she would, but instead of counting my blessings and being happy with that I decided to chance my arm, or in this case my ankle, and have another one done. As the new tattoo was on my ankle it would only be covered up when I wore jeans or a long skirt and that didn't happen very often. Subsequently, when Mum eventually found out, she chased me round the car! Boy, was I in trouble!

The only other incident I can think of that caused a similar amount of grief in our house was when I was caught smoking. Bearing in mind what I do for a living now that might well shock one or two people. It certainly did my mum. The thing is, my journey into

32

CrossFit hasn't been what you'd call orthodox. Especially when you compare me to the majority of other athletes.

Despite these rebellions, I still remained committed to trying loads of different sports as a teen. And with a typical teenage disregard to safety I was particularly attracted to sports that allowed you to work up a bit of speed. It was unsurprising, therefore, that sooner or later I was going to take up an activity that involved wheels. Up to this point, the only sport that I'd been involved in that had wheels attached to it was roller hockey, but when I was sixteen I discovered a new passion: cross-country mountain biking – or XC racing, as it's called.

As with roller hockey, it was speed that first attracted me to the sport and because I already enjoyed cross-country running it ticked a couple of boxes. Paul and I had had bikes since we were toddlers and given my love of sport, not to mention what we used to get up to at the farm next to my grandparents' house, it was all to be expected really. In fact, I'm surprised it didn't happen a bit sooner.

Speaking of Grandma and Grandad's house, one day the farm next door was broken into and the thieves took all the bikes and quad bikes. Although my grandparents didn't own the farm, some of the bikes that were taken belonged to us, and when the insurance money came through it was decided that, as opposed to replacing like for like, I'd get a nice shiny new mountain bike instead. I forget how much it cost exactly but it was around about my birthday time so with that taken into consideration we were able to buy a pretty hi-spec bike. It had front suspension, hundreds of gears and it looked fantastic.

The person who turned me onto XC racing was a boy from school who I also used to do karate with. After telling him about my new bike (I told everybody!), he told me all about XC racing and suggested I enter some races with him. I was so excited at the prospect of this, which is the effect sport usually has on me. This was slightly different, though, as the elements of danger and excitement would be magnified – and there's nothing I love more than a bit of danger and excitement. In fact, one usually leads to the other with me.

It's the same with theme parks. From as early as I can remember I was always the one who wanted to go on the biggest and fastest rollercoasters and, if I was too small to be allowed to go on one, I'd be beside myself. When I did get on I did so in the hope that I would be scared half to death and if I was surrounded by people screaming their heads off and being sick, then all the better. In fact, the only thing that I could have improved about those experiences, apart from making the rollercoasters bigger, of course, was to have been driving them myself. So, although the tracks and vehicles were a tiny bit smaller with XC racing, it was these same principles that attracted me: the danger was ever-present and I was in charge!

What surprised me most about the new bike was how light it was and, because it was so agile, I was able to more than satisfy my need for speed. It was brilliant. When I said that danger was ever-present I meant it, and had I continued competing into my twenties I doubt very much whether I'd have made it to my thirties. Certainly not in one piece.

The accidents themselves were all part and parcel. What used to annoy me was having to mend the bike. Or, worse still, not being able to mend the bike! That was a complete pain in the neck, as not only did it mean I couldn't carry on racing, but it meant I had to carry the bike and, depending on where I was, that could be a long way. My worst experience in this situation happened quite early on in my XC career and about two miles from the finish line. Because of my mentality, I refused to let a little thing like not having a working bike affect me as it might do any normal person, and, after crashing heavily at about thirty miles an hour and buckling one of my wheels, I jumped up, brushed myself down, picked up my bike and ran as fast as I possibly could to the finish line.

Although I joke about it, it was probably quite a pivotal moment for me really, as it was the first time I'd ever been in a situation where I had to make a decision as to whether I gave up or carried on. Although I obviously knew that I wasn't going to win the race, I was damned if I was going to just pack it in. So the only option open to me, and the only one I could have lived with myself for choosing, even at that age, was to carry on regardless and finish no matter what. I think it was also pivotal in that it was one of the first times Mum realised that just taking part wasn't good enough for me. I really did want it all!

A serious lust for danger notwithstanding, it was actually an injury that made me give up competing at XC racing. One day, we'd been training up on Harden Moor, which comprises woodland, several disused quarries and large stretches of heather. Perfect for XC racing. The training itself had gone really well but while cycling downhill into Keighley afterwards to get some lunch my front wheel locked up. Because we were on a road and not a track I wasn't expecting anything to happen and probably wasn't concentrating as much as I should have.

The accident happened in two parts. First, after my wheel locked up, I hit the kerb, which is when I realised that I might be in a bit of trouble. Part two had me smashing into a lamp post about a metre and a half from the kerb, which I remember hurting somewhat. It all happened in a flash, of course, although the memory of it happening is always in slow motion. After hitting the lamp post I then careered back onto the road where I slid down it about ten or fifteen metres before finally coming to a halt. It wasn't a very gracious descent, but as I said at the beginning, grace and poise have never been my strong points.

I didn't lose consciousness at first, but I was definitely a bit dazed and confused after it happened and for a few seconds I wasn't capable of moving. I was probably in shock. The guys I was with were ahead of me so didn't see me fall, which meant I was on my own. I managed to get myself onto the pavement where I actually did fall unconscious. Clearly someone must have seen me and raised the alarm, as next thing I knew I came round to see an ambulance parked up alongside me. The paramedics were in the process of putting me on the longboard (spine board) and loading me into the back of it.

Once I'd regained the power of speech I had one question for them.

'Where's my bike?' I asked in a panic.

'Never mind your bike,' said one of the paramedics. 'You've hurt yourself. Just sit back and try to relax, will you?'

'I can't relax. That bike cost a fortune! It's the most expensive thing I've ever had. We can't leave it!'

They were horrified when I asked if I could take it with me to the hospital.

'But what if somebody steals it?' I pleaded. 'It cost a fortune.'

'Couldn't one of your friends look after it for you?' countered a paramedic.

'No! It has to come with me.'

So much for relatives or friends accompanying people to hospital. Eventually the paramedics took pity and squeezed the battered frame into the back of the ambulance with me.

As well as splitting my helmet in two, I'd grazed most of my face, lost the majority of the skin on my chin and dislocated both my thumbs. I also had no skin left on either of my hips or my knees and had a selection of bruises that would have made a hundred peaches inedible. The soreness, though. That was so, so painful. And uncomfortable.

I was only in hospital a few hours and once again it was up to my grandma to come and get me.

'My word, you have been in the wars,' she said. 'Anyway, how's that expensive bike of yours?'

Spoken like a true Yorkshirewoman.

Despite the injuries, the reason I gave XC racing up after that was mainly because of timing – I had so much sport and studying going on while I was in the sixth form that it became too much to juggle. I knew I'd miss it, so the plan was always to go back next season when I wasn't as busy, but unfortunately that time didn't come. But I did do a couple of competitive XC races later on in life for the fire service.

The bike was not in good shape, by the way, and it took an awful lot of pocket money and odd-job money to supply it with various replacement parts. It probably took longer to recover than I did.

CHAPTER 5:

HERE COMES TROUBLE

I passed all of my GCSEs with good grades – so the world was my oyster. Or it would be, once I'd taken my A levels. For these, I decided to move schools as Pudsey Grangefield didn't do sports science, which was one of my chosen subjects. At this point I think I liked the idea of going down an academic route in my future career so, when I started my A levels, teaching was high up on the list. Until then my ambitions had gone from lawyer to truck driver, military to scientist, travel rep to doctor. Although it never lost me any sleep, it was a dilemma of sorts. Quite a nice one, though.

The biggest thing to happen in my life outside of sport and education when I started my A levels was discovering alcohol and nightclubs. The people I studied with were a bit more advanced in that department than I was and one of the first things they asked me when I started studying was if I fancied going into Leeds.

'What, you mean on a night out?' I asked innocently.

'Yeah, of course. We're all off to the Majestic tomorrow.'

I tried my best to remain cool but inside I was turning somersaults. I'd obviously been into Leeds before but never socially, and never after dark! The Majestic nightclub isn't there any more (in fact, it's the new headquarters of Channel 4) but the building is slap bang in the middle of the centre and at the time it was the best-known nightclub in the city. I'd heard about the Majestic, but had never even dreamt about going. Surely this meant adulthood was just around the corner?

Before committing fully to the trip I had to get permission from my mum, although I didn't tell my fellow pupils that. As far as they were concerned it was no big deal.

'Yeah, count me in,' I'd said to them, almost nonchalantly. 'It'll be a laugh.'

When I went to ask Mum I was petrified. She was never an especially strict parent, but she was also no fool and if she thought that going to the Majestic with some other seventeen-years-olds was beyond my experience she'd have no problem saying so. After all, I was technically still underage.

'What do you think, Andy?' she said, looking at my stepdad. 'It's a big step.'

They could have stopped the conversation there and then by reminding me that I was underage so they obviously must have trusted me.

'I'll tell you what,' said my stepdad. 'How about we agree to you going as long as I can pick you up?'

Some people would have been mortified by this – you know, the embarrassment – but to me it meant one thing: a free taxi!

'Yeah, okay then. Are you sure you don't mind coming out at that time?'

'If it'll stop your mother worrying and you're not sick on the car seats, then no, I don't mind at all.'

Going to the Majestic was a rite of passage for me – we ended up going on a fairly regular basis. Despite being seventeen I must have been one of the oldest people in that nightclub. I'd never seen

40

anything like it! When it came to the dancing part, I had to have a beer or two for some Dutch courage. Memories of ballet recitals were still fresh in the mind but once I was up there I was fine. Or at least I felt fine. God knows what I looked like.

Like a good girl, I always turned up at the agreed pick-up point every time Andy agreed to pick me up and was never once sick on the car seats. Well, not that I can remember. I was sick on Mum though, at least once. Again, I don't remember this, but she certainly does. I'd been home for about half an hour after being out when all of a sudden Mum heard a call from my room.

'Mum, I don't feel well,' I moaned.

'Come downstairs and I'll get you a glass of water,' she said. 'Did you have too much to drink?'

Apparently I walked to the bottom of the stairs where Mum was standing and before I could even reply to her question I answered it by vomiting on her shoes.

'That'll be a yes then,' she said.

'Sorry, Mum. I feel ill!'

My poor mother. She had a lot to put up with when it came to me. My main character trait when I was young (Mum would probably call it a flaw) was being mischievous. By the time I was in my teens I was an absolute menace and I treated pranking almost like a sport. When I went to ask Mum for some material for the book she put together a list of examples. Or, in her words, 'What not to do when you're around Sam Briggs':

1. *Don't, whatever you do, bend over in front of an open cupboard to put your boots on when Sam's standing behind you.* This refers to the time I pushed my mum into a cupboard, closed the door and walked off. Unfortunately, Mum doesn't seem

to learn by her mistakes as this has happened quite a few times and probably will again. Well, hopefully.

2. *Don't leave the door unlocked when you're in the bath and Sam's nearby.* This one refers to the time I opened the bathroom door slightly, reached in and turned off the light. Needless to say, there was a lot of splashing around and a lot of bad language coming from the bathroom afterwards.

3. *Don't trust Sam Briggs with condiments at Nando's.* I love chicken, but what I love even more than chicken is smothering my mum's meal in the hottest Peri-Peri sauce Nando's have to offer. That one didn't go down so well.

4. *Don't fall asleep when Sam Briggs has a pen in her hand.* Being a frustrated tattooist, I'm always on the lookout for guinea pigs, conscious or unconscious. So, if I see somebody asleep who has skin, and most people do, the chances are I'll draw something on it. Again, this has happened more than once and the first time I did it was on Mum's face. I wish I could remember what it was. It was detailed, that's all I remember. Another time I drew the leaning tower of Pisa on one of her legs and a smiley face on the other. I absolutely love drawing on skin and if Mum wasn't asleep I'd just keep on asking her until she said yes. 'Can I draw on you? Can I draw on you?' It was pure pester power.

5. *If you're going away on holiday make sure you lock your wardrobe or take all your clothes with you.* After all, there's nothing worse than receiving photographs of your dog wearing all your best gear when you're lying on a beach, is there?

6. *Don't let Sam give you a massage.* As a child I became a budding masseuse and Mum was happy to let me practise on her – she worked long hours and, when she finally came

home, she was usually exhausted and would welcome a back rub. 'Here, Mum,' I'd say. 'Why don't you lie down on your bed and I'll practise on you?' I don't know why but one day I got bored of massaging Mum with baby oil, so I swapped it for yogurt and a sprinkle of cornflakes. Mum was so tired she didn't notice at first, so I just carried on. 'How's that for you?' I said. 'All right?'

'Ooh, that's lovely, Sam.'

I think it was when I poured more cornflakes on that Mum twigged what was going on and when I told her that I'd been massaging her with yogurt and breakfast cereal she hit the roof. Understandably, I suppose. She hates waste.

7. *Do not allow Sam Briggs to rid you of a cyst.* This one's awful! About three years before I started using dairy products and cereals as massage lubricants, Mum developed a cyst on her forehead. She'd never had anything like it before in her life and was horrified when it arrived. Ever the dutiful daughter, I told Mum that I'd read up on how to remove cysts and, if she left it to me, I'd get rid of it for her. My mum is a really bright woman but on this particular occasion she'd obviously given her brain a day off. As opposed to going to the doctors she told me to carry on and then asked me what I was going to do. 'The best way to get rid of cysts,' I began, 'is to hit them with a Bible.' Once again Mum's brain failed to engage and after being instructed to commence with the treatment I found a Bible, told Mum to shut her eyes and then gave the cyst an almighty whack. Or a whack from the Almighty, you might say.

Unfortunately, my course of treatment, which I think I'd got from a book about witchcraft, resulted in Mum needing to have surgery! I think I'd got the witchcraft book from my grandad. He was always mad about ghost stories, so I was weaned on them. Them and horror films. Not my finest hour.

Something else not many people know about me is that I have extremely dexterous toes. It doesn't really help with CrossFit unfortunately (or it hasn't yet) but it makes people laugh. I can pick up all kinds of random objects with my toes and can even pick up a pencil and start drawing with it. I don't know why I included that! Let's get back to the story …

CHAPTER 6:

FINDING THE RIGHT PATH

The subjects I took for A level were maths with statistics, sports science and biology. Although I worked hard for my A levels, I didn't put in the effort I should have to achieve the grades I was capable of. In hindsight I probably should have taken this as a sign that academia just wasn't for me, but instead I decided to continue with my studies and accepted a place at Leeds University where I was due to read maths with biology.

Once again, I think I liked the idea of being in academia, and anybody who's been to university (or anyone who hasn't, come to think of it) will probably agree that the prospect of spending three years having fun with your mates, drinking your own bodyweight in alcohol every night and going to the odd lecture isn't a bad one. Unfortunately, that wasn't the reality for me.

After I left school, a lot of the teams I'd been involved in had either stopped or were no longer relevant to somebody my age, and during my A levels that situation had become worse. It was my own fault, I suppose, as I allowed it to slip, but by the time I went to university I had a job working in a bar and had given up sport altogether. It's hard to believe looking back but it's true. Apathy and alcohol had got the better of me. As opposed to starting university, like I had school, with a hundred and one activities to do, I was spending all of my time in the bar either working, drinking or both. I was eating badly and most days I woke up with a hangover so I was never in the mood for anything really, least of all studying or sitting in a lecture hall and certainly not playing sport. I expect this happens to lots of students but I didn't realise how much I'd let myself go and how much I needed to be fit. Without any physical activity to perk me up I was just tired and bleary-eyed all the time. I'd gone from being one of the world's most active people (well, in my head) to one of the world's most inactive within a matter of months and it had left me totally flat.

I think some people assume that I've been a tower of strength and motivation since birth, but in reality I've experienced both sides of the coin. That said, regardless of how much life changes you can always pull yourself back. In order to kick-start my life again I knew I'd have to make wholesale changes, beginning with deciding what I wanted to do for a living. I knew that I was getting into a bad rut and things couldn't go on as they were.

I should point out, by the way, that, despite the realisation that I was in the wrong place both physically and mentally, I did have a really good time at university, in that I met some amazing people, had a few drinks and laughed a lot. I certainly wasn't crying myself to sleep every night, nor was I moping around feeling sorry for myself. But the feeling of dissatisfaction was like an itch that I desperately needed to scratch. A big one!

Had I gone public with my feelings as soon as I started having them I'd have been out of university and back home within about half a day. But of course there was a bit more to consider in the bigger picture and I didn't want to let anyone down, so instead of just packing up and running home immediately I decided to leave it and give it more time. That was probably the apathy talking too, to be honest, but I also needed to pluck up the courage to tell everyone – and telling people you've made a big mistake and are ultimately a bit unhappy isn't always easy. What compounded this was the realisation that, from now on, every day spent at university was effectively a day wasted and, as you already know, I do not like wasting time.

The catalyst for me finally picking up the phone and calling it a day happened when I went to buy a pair of jeans one day. I'd been wearing Levi's for most of my later teen years and buying a new pair of jeans was normally a formality. Go to the shop, choose a pair, try them on just in case and then get your money out. Simple. What had gradually been happening though was I'd be having to buy a bigger size each time – no big deal, probably just this style! However, this time was different. In the changing rooms I thought I must have picked up the wrong size or something, but no, I hadn't. I now couldn't fit into any of the styles of my once-loved jeans. The old jeans I'd been wearing had obviously been stretched to the hilt and I remember thinking to myself, *God, what's happened to me?*

I knew something had to change. I wasn't happy studying and somewhere along the way I had lost all my motivation. The jeans incident was the moment when I realised just how much I'd let myself go and how much I needed to be physically active again to get back on track.

I certainly wasn't the first student to realise that university wasn't for them and I obviously wouldn't be the last, but the relief I felt when I finally made the call was massive. Just talking about it and admitting that I'd made a mistake and needed to make a change was amazing. When I picked up the phone to call Mum I had butterflies in my stomach the size of bats, but not because I thought she'd be angry or disappointed. Mum's always wanted me and Paul to be happy, end of story, and I think she was concerned by the fact that I was drinking a lot and wasn't playing sport. It was just the significance of what the telephone call meant really – that is, me leaving university early and ultimately being free to do something that would hopefully make me happy.

The effect that leaving university and giving up the job in the bar had on my life was immediate. It was like a breath of fresh air. For the first time in months I felt alive. Instead of waking up in the morning, turning over and going back to sleep again, which had become the normality, I was out of bed and doing something active within minutes. It didn't matter what it was or where, I just didn't want to be in bed.

Although I've never regretted my decision to choose a more physical profession over an academic one, I do get the urge sometimes to go back and revisit that side of things. When I was in the fire service, I did actually go back to university to take an evening class in business administration. With age comes experience, and because I obviously know more about life now than I did twenty years ago, my appetite to learn and, latterly, become more involved in CrossFit has expanded. For instance, over the last few years I've been reading a lot of books about sports psychology. Textbooks and papers mainly. As a subject it piques my interest and I wouldn't bet against me doing an Open University degree one day. If I ever get time.

But for now it was such a joy to reconnect with my physical fitness and to get active and start moving again. So it was perfect timing when, just a few days after I left university, a friend of mine who played for Bradford City Women's Football Club called me up. She knew I was wanting to get fit again and the ladies' second team was looking for players so she suggested I started training to try out for the team.

Had she called me a fortnight earlier I'd probably have found an excuse not to do it. That was it, you see; while I was at university I could easily have joined a football team or gone to a gym, but something seemed to stop me. The bar, mainly! Not any more, though. I was now free from all that and it was time for me to take on a new challenge. Having an addictive personality is great when it is focused on something like sport; if I'm not trying to be the best at something physical, then, as we found out, I'd try to be the best at things not so productive like drinking, and I'm definitely a better person when I'm focusing on sport!

After taking part in a couple of training sessions I was asked if I'd like to play a match for the Bradford City ladies' second team. In terms of what I'd been aiming for post university this was the first rung of the ladder and I was absolutely thrilled to bits. I was part of a team again, and gradually I lost the weight and regained my fitness. The second rung was obviously playing for the first team, which came several months later. From then on there was no stopping me. It wasn't like I was playing professional football – for cup games we used to get a fee of around £10 – but it was exactly what I needed and I loved being back. If we'd been in it solely for the money we'd have starved!

I played for Bradford for a long time but as I was getting older there were fewer opportunities to play for the first team, so a friend suggested I try out for a rival team called Leeds City Vixens. They too were in the Northern Premier League and I had played against them before with Bradford. Changing teams was the best move for me and I ended up playing four very happy seasons with them.

Leeds City Vixens are now called Leeds City, having merged with Abbey Grange FC and Adel FC, and one of the biggest games I played for them was against Leeds United ladies. It was a County Cup match and, despite being a Leeds United supporter (I was given no choice as a child!), I was looking forward to it. There was a big mention in the press; with it being a derby match the game had attracted quite a bit of attention. Leeds United were clear favourites to win the game and all the talk in the press and on the forums said that we were going to get crushed.

Crushed or not, I was going to enjoy the experience no matter what and, when we turned up for the match at Thorp Arch, Leeds United's training ground, we were more than a little excited. We knew they were good and we were the underdogs, so we had nothing to lose and everything to gain. Instead of arguing with people or even getting involved in conversations about it, we agreed to do our talking on the pitch. Had we been expecting a big defeat then perhaps we'd have joined in with the fun, but the fact is, we weren't. From the first whistle we took the game to Leeds and I think the shock almost paralysed them. They did settle down after a while, but we were well in control by then and they never made it back. We beat them 2–1, but it should have been 4.

On the flipside of that, we once played Scunthorpe United ladies' team at their training ground and about halfway through the first half our goalkeeper got injured. I didn't think for a moment that they'd ask me to replace her so when the coaches were busy deliberating I just sat on the touchline and had a drink.

'Sam, would you come over here please?' one of them said finally.

'Yep, sure.'

It still hadn't occurred to me that I was about to be moved back a few positions and when the coach asked me I was speechless.

'Is there nobody else?' I asked.

As I spoke, I tried thinking of a team-mate who might fare better between the sticks. Then it occurred to me that by suggesting somebody else I might appear cowardly, so without waiting for an answer I said quickly, 'Don't worry, I'll do it.'

'Thanks, Sam,' said the coach. 'Here's some gloves. Go and have a quick word with your team.'

Not only was it a really important match but the last time I'd played in goal was probably during a roller-hockey game on our street at least a decade ago and that fact wasn't lost on me. In fact, it was all I could think about!

Doing as the coach said, I put on my gloves and called the team around me for a chat. I was so, so nervous.

'Right then, you lot,' I began. 'It's your job to stop Scunthorpe from shooting. Do you understand? This isn't my usual position and I want you to do everything in your power to prevent me from having to handle the ball!'

I don't think the speech inspired much confidence in my team. They just stood there looking confused and a bit nervous. Needless to say, we lost the match and by quite some margin. These days I only wear gloves to keep the cold out. Never, ever again!

CHAPTER 7:

SIGNING UP FOR SERVICE

When I decided that I was going to leave university, there were three professions I had in mind: the RAF, the police force and the fire service. In truth, the three had been on my mind long before I even applied to go to university and if I had my time again I'd probably spend some of it exploring the opportunities within the three services. The one that always attracted me the most was the fire service. There used to be a television programme when I was a kid called *London's Burning* and, although it didn't glamorise the profession exactly, it used to highlight the other more truthful and attractive aspects to the job, such as the camaraderie. The idea of being a good team player really used to resonate with me, and I used to dream about what it would be like to be a firefighter.

Without wanting to sound too virtuous, I also wanted to put something back into society and, although all three services obviously ticked that particular box, the fire service seemed to be a little bit more 'me'. Giving something back had been at the forefront of my mind while I was applying for university too, and I'd been intending to fulfil it by becoming a teacher. I wonder how that would have worked out? I think I'd have been okay.

To hedge my bets, I did actually apply to join all three services when I left university, although I withdrew my application from the

RAF quite early on. I think Mum would have had a heart attack had I joined the RAF so to save me from any awkward conversations I decided to put my efforts into the other two. Had I been as keen on the RAF as I was on the fire service, it might have been a different matter, but it just didn't grab me enough.

I got through to the interview stage with both the police and the fire service and when it was finally time to choose between the two I stuck with my original choice. Everybody likes firefighters, right? Being accepted into the West Yorkshire Fire and Rescue Service was a huge honour and it's still a great source of pride for me. I felt like I'd achieved something massive when I got the news, and the anticipation I felt prior to starting my training was similar to how I felt when I arrived at my first CrossFit Games back in (oh my God, was it really?) 2010.

The process of me actually joining the fire service was rather protracted, as halfway through some budget cuts came in, which meant my application was put on hold. I had to wait just under a year for the process to start again but I never once thought about ditching it and doing something else. Budget cuts or not, we're always going to need a fire service and the longer I had to wait the more I looked forward to it. Altogether, with initial applications, applications on hold, testing and interviews, it took almost two years to get in.

After finally being accepted in 2004, I had to go on a three-month residential training course. I don't know what it's like these days but I'm pretty sure that firefighters just train during the day and are free to return home at night. But give me a residential course any day of the week. I loved it! It was very regimental, and we were bossed around and shouted at from dawn until dusk. Every morning our beds and kit would be inspected and if everything

54

wasn't exactly as it should be you were in big trouble. On Friday night when you were allowed to go home it was like, yes, freedom! Then on Sunday when you had to go back again you were a bit more subdued. That said, once you were there and all together again it was fine. Although I've never been in the army, I'm assuming it's a similar process to theirs and the clichés are correct, it is character building. Or at least it was for me.

Although we'd been accepted and were training, we were still very much on probation and if you didn't cut the mustard at any point throughout the three months you were either chucked out completely, or, if they thought you still had potential, you were back-coursed, which means being sent home initially but then given a place on the next course. It was brutal stuff, looking back.

There were certain weeks where beasting was the name of the game – in the first week we lost one recruit, but the hardest weeks were week three and four where the majority were either back-coursed or thrown out. The parts I found the most enjoyable during those early weeks were the really difficult ones like running with hoses and carrying ladders. Despite being integral to the job, these skills were alien to us all, which meant that everybody was starting from scratch. The ladders we used were called 135s and, as well as having an extended length of 13.5 metres (the clue's in the name, I suppose), they weighed over 100kg. We had to go over an assault course carrying one of these as a team so as well as being fit you also had to be strong and agile.

A few hours after completing the course, I heard that three recruits had been back-coursed in that one day. I wasn't at all surprised. Everyone had struggled a bit and it had obviously exposed some weaknesses.

Because so many recruits had been back-coursed at once, the officer in charge of equalities came down from headquarters and apparently he was in a right flap.

'You can't possibly get rid of the only female we have on the training course,' he said to the instructors. 'It's not on!'

'What do you mean?' they replied.

'I heard you had to let three go,' said the officer, 'so I came straight down. I assume she's one of them.'

'You mean Sam? No, she passed with flying colours.'

I'm afraid the equalities officer had had a wasted journey. It was kind of him to think of me, though.

I won't pretend I didn't get any satisfaction from that, because I did. Just a bit. But I'd had to work hard for it. Really hard.

I remember on a couple of occasions they kept us up all night during the training course but rather than just sitting around we were kept physically and mentally busy the whole time. I remember thinking to myself, *What the heck's this all about?* A few months later the reason became apparent, as sometimes as a firefighter you get evenings when you literally don't have time to sit down. Because of the responsibility you have to yourself, your colleagues and the public, it's imperative that you can remain alert and handle the situation.

When the three months were up, we had a passing-out parade at the West Yorkshire Fire and Rescue headquarters which are in Birkenshaw, Bradford. This is where all the square bashing we'd done at the start of the course came in useful, as we had to wear our best dress kit and march up and down a lot in front of our families and friends. You could see your face in my shoes.

When talking about my time in the fire service, people often ask if I experienced any sexism or sexist behaviour and the truth is I never did. I also didn't experience any preferential treatment which, to be honest, would have annoyed me just as much. At my first station, which was in a place called Morley, near Leeds, I was the first female firefighter they'd ever had working there, so on my arrival they were a little uncertain as to how things would be, but I just wanted to be treated like everyone else so I slotted in perfectly. Okay, the only preferential treatment I received was when it came to working night shifts. There was a dormitory full of beds but without even asking they felt I'd rather have my own room and gave me the crew manager's room. Fortunately, my enthusiasm for becoming one of the lads was outweighed slightly by a hunch that, should I have to share a dormitory with a load of hefty blokes, I may encounter a certain amount of snoring. So if I wanted to get my beauty sleep, I'd be far better off saying thanks very much and having my own dorm, albeit with just one bed in it. My hunch ended up paying dividends because some of the noises that used to emanate from that dormitory were like something out of a horror film!

My stay at Morley Fire Station lasted a year, which was the length of my probation. After that you were allowed to put in for a transfer and you had to give them a list of three stations you'd like to go to. Mine were Leeds, Bradford and Hunslet, which is in south Leeds but covers some of the centre. The reason I chose those three was because, unlike Morley, they were busy multi-pump stations; being young and enthusiastic I wanted to be where the action was and get as much experience as was humanly possible. In the end, I was given my first choice of Hunslet, which meant I was really in the thick of it. At Morley there'd been only four of us on shift, whereas at Hunslet there were at least twelve. This time, though, there was no female dormitory, so instead of being able to retire to my own room in silence I had to lie there and pray that the snoring started after I'd gone to sleep.

The wage jump after passing your probation was massive and the first thing I did after completing it was to go out and buy a sports car. As stated, I'm somewhat of a speed freak and in the months leading up to me being a fully fledged firefighter the prospect of me becoming mobile with something that was a little bit nippier than a pushbike or a fire engine was tantalising. In the end I got myself a gorgeous little second-hand Honda S2000 and, my word, it was fast. Unfortunately, it was also thirsty!

Next on my post-probation to-do list was to move to a new house. Because I hadn't been earning very much I'd decided to move back in with Mum and Andy and, although I'd enjoyed it, I was looking forward to having my own space again. Within a week of me moving out, the reality of running a sports car and a flat started to hit home and a month later I sold the car. I couldn't actually afford to put petrol in it so, although it looked nice parked outside the flat, it was useless. It was fun while I had it, though. These days I drive a Mini which is just as nippy as the Honda was but a lot less thirsty.

Until then I'd always had a topsy-turvy relationship with money and had gone through several stages of being careful, followed by frivolous. One of these had resulted in me getting into a little bit of a debt and, after being coached (that's another word for being ticked off) by my mum about how to manage my finances, I thought I'd got it out of my system. I remember the time well. I'd just turned eighteen and had learned that banks were willing to give me lots of money. Lots of spending money! Unfortunately, the bit I hadn't listened to was that one day I'd have to pay the money back and when that time finally came it was all a bit of a shock. *You mean you want the money back? With interest? That's outrageous!* It took me a while but after keeping all the local petrol stations in profit for a few months I'd finally learned the error of my ways. Now with a new house, a more sensible car and an exciting new job, I felt I was back on the path to happiness.

CHAPTER 8:

LIFE ON THE FRONTLINE

One of the main considerations for me when choosing to join the fire service had been how fit you had to be – and how fit you had to continue being. This was also taken into account when choosing Hunslet as my first proper station, as with more firefighters present I figured there'd be more opportunities to play sport and train. Fortunately, I was right. During our physical training sessions, which we had several times a week, we'd go down to South Leeds Stadium, which is just down the road from the station, and play five-a-side football. Once again, I was given no preferential treatment whatsoever by my male counterparts, and with no mercy being shown by anyone on the pitch I was able to play a very fast and physical game. I remember being floored on several occasions by our station manager! It was excellent.

In between night shifts, some of us would go out on our mountain bikes for the day and if you take into account the time we all spent in the gym, which was a lot, you could say that from a physical point of view I'd landed on my feet. It was a far, far cry from my months at university and, because I was now able to buy a new pair of jeans again without wanting the floor to swallow me up, I couldn't have been happier.

The main downside to working as a firefighter are some of the things you witness either during or after fires. It's something you can read and hear about until you're blue in the face, but you can never really prepare yourself for it. Unfortunately, it's a part of the job you have to experience first-hand in order to learn how to handle it and some do that better than others.

The first house fire I ever attended was in an upstairs flat. After finding an unconscious survivor in one of the bedrooms I had to pick them up and then carry them to safety as quickly as I could. Although they were still alive at the time, the victim had suffered some dreadful burns and, when I tried to move their arms in order to be able to lift them, skin started peeling off. That was a huge and horrible shock and, again, it's not something you can easily prepare for. The only thing that mattered at the time was the person I was trying to help and, regardless of how gruesome and upsetting the situation was, I had an opportunity to move them and get them to safety so I just had to get on with it.

Once outside, the paramedics got to work and after several minutes trying they managed to revive the poor soul, but only momentarily. Given the burns they'd suffered, perhaps that was the best outcome. Either way, it was an event that I had to try to process quickly and fortunately I found that quite easy. Not because I didn't care about what had happened; I obviously did. It was the realisation that, if I couldn't learn to handle seeing something like that, I'd be no use as a firefighter, and as somebody who's always been a very practical person that wasn't an option.

I remember arriving home that night after my shift had ended. After telling Mum what had happened, she gave me my tea and then sat down with me at the table.

'Do you want to talk about it, Sam?' she asked. 'It must have been harrowing for you.'

I think I was already halfway through my tea by this point. You see, practical.

The only events that ever stayed with me were those involving children and I think that's the same with all firefighters, regardless of your natural disposition or experience. The worst one I ever attended happened just before Christmas one year. I was covering for somebody over in Bradford and at about 10 p.m. we were called out to an RTC (road traffic collision). The one car involved had three people inside: a young teenage boy who'd been driving and two teenage passengers, a boy in the front and a girl in the back. Apparently they'd been joyriding and, as so often happens in these situations, the driver had lost control. The only one to escape the accident was the boy in the front seat, whereas the other two didn't make it. As we cut them out of the wreckage, all I could think about were the families of these kids and what kind of effect it would have on them. Not just now, but for the rest of their lives. I also thought about the police officers who were going to have to give them the news. The part we had to play wasn't exactly a walk in the park but imagine having to do that.

One of the things that firefighters are most famous for, although it's a bit of an urban myth really, is rescuing kittens from trees. The closest I got to one of those call-outs was rescuing one from a car engine, which I think is far more original. I was working at Stanningley Fire Station at the time and we got a call from a woman who had turned her engine on before realising, fortunately very quickly, that there was something under the bonnet that shouldn't have been there. Because I was always the smallest person on the watch, if we ever had to enter a small space I'd be one to go, although I have to confess that climbing into the workings of a car was a new one.

The poor kitten, who had been a little bit too inquisitive for its own good, had got one of its paws caught in the fanbelt as the woman had started her engine and it was lucky not to have been seriously injured or even killed. As you know, I absolutely adore animals and, as I went to try to extract the poor thing, I was full of concern and sympathy. About a minute later, as the kitten was scratching the hell out of my hands, wrists and forearms, my sympathy for the animal had started to wane a little bit and my whispers of, 'Hello, little man, don't worry, I've come to help,' were replaced with pain-filled cries of, 'Ow! You evil little sod! I'm trying to help you, for heaven's sake!' When I finally managed to get hold of the little devil and untangled its paw from the fanbelt I took several more scratches before removing it from the car and presenting it to his worried owner. 'There you are,' I said through gritted teeth. 'One slightly damaged kitten.' As I handed the kitten to its owner I looked down at my hand and forearm and it was like something out of a slasher movie! Gosh, that was painful.

Another quite amusing story from my time as a firefighter involves us being called out to a chemical spill one day. It might sound a bit strange but when we first arrived at the scene it was actually quite impressive, as the colours of the chemicals, which had spilled onto some concrete before interspersing, were amazing. There were also a few bangs happening here and there, so it was like a liquid firework display. The first thing we did after arriving was to ask the company whose premises we were attending if any of the chemicals were dangerous. Although colourful, they certainly looked potentially hazardous, and we were all a bit wary. After about half an hour our boss appeared, having been assured by the company that all was well, so we got to work.

About two hours into the job, however, somebody noticed an unusual issue: it seemed their boots were starting to melt! A quarter of an hour later, everyone was suffering the same problem. I remember sitting in the engine having been ordered to remove myself from the scene and my boots were literally falling off my feet! who knows what the chemicals were but the company who called us out had to foot the bill (pardon the pun) for about twenty pairs of boots.

When it comes to being scared, there's only one contender with regards to stories from my time in the fire service and again it involves chemicals. We were called out to a fire at a chemical plant one day and when we arrived there were hundreds of metal canisters lining the floor of a warehouse. With the fire not being that far away it was imperative that we kept these canisters cool and there must have been at least twenty of us, all on different lines, trying to do just that. We had no idea what was in these canisters, which made the situation even more precarious. Whilst cooling the canisters the fire engulfed some other containers up front, causing a huge explosion. This created what's called a flame front, which is a region of space where combustion takes place. Or, in layman's terms, a huge blue and green flame that in this case was almost as wide as the warehouse and was moving very quickly in our direction.

Fortunately, the flame front was about five feet off the ground so, after throwing ourselves down as fast as we possibly could (it was like a very quick game of musical bumps), we turned onto our backs, aimed our hoses skywards and hoped for the best. It can't have lasted more than about ten seconds but it seemed like ten minutes. I remember hearing a lot of nervous laughter and nobody moved a muscle for about three minutes after the flame subsided. I think we were all in shock.

Obviously most days in the fire service weren't quite as memorable or traumatic as these but it really was an incredible job and I was learning something new every day. One of the great things about it was that you had room to grow in the role. Because I'd gained good grades at school and had flirted with university, the powers that be at the fire service asked me one day if I'd be interested in going for a management position.

'What would that entail?' I asked.

'Initially, it would mean you having to take a few exams,' replied my boss. 'Then, if you pass those exams, you'll be able to provide cover for absent crew commanders. It would mean extra money and extra responsibility.'

After he made it clear to me that it would just be a few hours a week over a period of months as opposed to something intense, I agreed to give it a go. Not only because I liked the idea of potentially furthering my career, but because I knew I had it in me to do something that put my brain to good use and the fact that it wouldn't be to the detriment of my fitness or physicality sealed the deal.

There was a lot of work to do, but I was motivated and interested, and I passed the exams with flying colours. After covering for crew commanders for a year or so, I was asked if I'd like to take my crew commander's exams, and, having enjoyed filling in, I jumped at the chance. Being able to dip my toe in the water had allowed me to enjoy studying again, so, although going for crew commander would mean ramping things up a level, I was satisfied that it would still be okay. As this was happening

I was approached by a team from head office who were scouting for people with high potential (it sounds dangerously like hypertension when you say it quickly!) and to cut a long story short they ended up putting me on a fast-track scheme that would hopefully take me through the promotions. Even with this going on, I didn't feel daunted, as I'd established myself in the sports I was practising and was managing my time a lot more efficiently. It was a really good time to be alive.

After becoming a crew commander, I was in training to become a watch commander. As part of that development, I worked as watch commander at head office in resilience planning, making emergency plans for if major incidents or terrorist action happened. After completing that training, I was assigned my own watch at a one-pump station. I was there for a year before being assigned to a multi-pump station which, in terms of incidents, meant that I was able to be in charge of call-outs that had up to three pumps present. This was the big league.

One thing I was conscious of in the fire service was trying to avoid being a token woman and that's one of the things that pushed me to move up through the ranks and keep on improving. This wasn't a feminist struggle as such; it was a personal one. A competitive and determined human being wanting to prove to themselves that they're as good and as capable as anyone else. What also drove me on was the fact that I enjoyed both sides of my job – the physical and the managerial side – so I was motivated to do well in both and I was able to hold my own with everyone I worked with. The more I pushed myself the better I became, and the only way to get better still was to diversify and to keep challenging myself.

I'm running away a little here, but that's the ethos behind CrossFit really and, in terms of having a job that would, by default of course, prepare me for life as a CrossFit athlete, the fire service was perfect. Hard work, camaraderie and an ability to cope with anything life throws at you – those three things are at the heart of the fire service and they're at the heart of CrossFit too.

CHAPTER 9:

SPORTING LIFE

In 2008, I decided to move to Manchester and, although I was able to remain with the West Yorkshire Fire Service and commute, I decided to move football teams. My new team, Curzon and Ashton FC, were based in Ashton-under-Lyne and they had a really good setup. I was looking forward to it.

However, just a few weeks after joining the team I was playing a five-a-side match one day when I injured my ankle. Because I didn't really know the people I was playing with very well I just hobbled off and went home, and after a rubbish night's sleep I woke up to find that my foot and ankle were twice their normal size. Somehow I managed to get myself to work and after spending twenty-five minutes trying to squeeze my foot and ankle into my boot I decided there and then to retire from playing football permanently. It wasn't a tough decision, although I was certainly going to miss it. My job came first and, if I had to take time off every time I had an injury, I'd be letting an awful lot of people down. It's not that I was an irresponsible person prior to joining the fire service, but my sense of responsibility post joining definitely changed, and I became far more mature.

With no football to keep me occupied, I had to find something else to do, and quickly. It's like having a dog. If you don't exercise them regularly, they go bonkers and I was definitely no different. In the end I decided to join a running club and the nearest one to me in Manchester was Salford. The main problem with football as far as I was concerned was obviously the contact, so, although my career in running was unlikely to be injury-free, at least I wouldn't have four or ten other people trying to tackle me. My ankle in particular had taken a real battering over the years and I was constantly going over on it and spraining it. It was no fun.

Fortunately, running very soon became a direct replacement for football and as well as keeping me very fit the social side was excellent, as it enabled me to meet new people. I'd also joined a gym over in Manchester, obviously, and that too had been a godsend in terms of helping me settle into the area. Something else that kept me occupied, apart from firefighting, running, mountain biking (which I still did in between night shifts with the boys from work) and attending a gym five or six times a week, was swimming. It was the boys at work who'd convinced me to try triathlons, but I needed to work on my swimming first. In truth I was probably okay; I was just very inefficient and used my arms way too much, so I dedicated time to that.

I did try my hand at synchronised swimming once. I'd forgotten about that! I was probably only about twelve or thirteen at the time and the reason I gave it a go was to help my breathing under water, and then Mum got roped into teaching it. Why she used to teach it I absolutely have no idea. She'd never done it herself. I think it was one of those situations where the regular teacher left and because it was a kids' class they just went with any parent who was willing to blag it. Sorry, I meant teach it! It was the blind leading the blind, basically. Anyway, because Mum was now teaching the classes I had to keep going and it's probably one of the few times in my life when I've done a sport not to hurt somebody's feelings. Well, that and the fact that I was keen to improve my breathing under water.

Bearing in mind what I've already told you about the ballet, it perhaps won't surprise you to learn that synchronised swimming was not my cup of tea. According to Mum, my downfall in the sport – this is in addition to a complete lack of skill, control, technique and poise – was my refusal to wear a nose clip. I genuinely don't remember this, but Mum says I was always resolute and regardless of how many times she pleaded with me the answer was always no. She also says that because I wouldn't wear a nose clip I always came out of the water coughing and spluttering, which is why I was never selected to appear at any exhibitions. Well, that and the fact that I couldn't actually do it! Sam Briggs, synchronised swimmer. No, it just doesn't work. I don't think I've ever told anyone about this, so I have no idea why I'm putting it in here. It seems mad really.

So back to why the boys at work had started pushing me towards swimming and us starting to dabble in triathlons. This quickly became the main reason for them encouraging me to improve my swimming, so it was straight down to the pool for me and no arguments. Given what I've already said about being able to turn my hand to different sports and disciplines – and enjoying it, of course – competing in a triathlon seemed like a natural progression, and the fact that there were several of us from the fire station taking part and training together made it feel almost like a team sport. Not unlike CrossFit, I suppose.

I remember my first triathlon as clear as day, and, surprise surprise, the only part I had any trouble with was the open water swim. Being a strong and confident swimmer is obviously a necessity with triathlons, regardless of the distance you're doing. I'd certainly improved by this time but not to a point where I was particularly confident. Sure enough, almost from the start, I had people pulling my legs and trying to swim over me. It was awful!

Despite it being a baptism of fire, I'm so glad it happened, as ultimately it has helped me to prepare for the mass starts we sometimes have at the CrossFit Games. These feature both the men and the women and as you can imagine they're absolute carnage. Nobody gives anybody any quarter whatsoever and weaker or less confident swimmers are found out very, very quickly. I think the last time we had one of these was in 2015 and, despite me being light years ahead of where I was in 2008, which is when I started working on my swimming again, I still ended up almost drowning! Okay, that might be a bit of an exaggeration but it's not far off.

The race started on a beach in California and after completing a 50-metre sprint we had a 200-metre swim ahead of us followed by a 50-metre sprint at the other end. On paper it doesn't sound too difficult but when you take into account who you're racing against you start considering factors such as intensity. This was about survival!

Sure enough, when we got into the water it was aquatic chaos on a grand scale and my nemesis throughout the entire swim was one Spencer Hendel. As well as being about 8 feet tall, Spencer's quite broad and his legs and arms are probably about the same length as my entire person. Consequently, when Spencer first decided to swim over me there was nothing I could do about it, as with Triathlon there are no rules stating you can't swim over the other athletes, so Spencer was taking full advantage of this. When I managed to get past him again (I think I went around him as opposed to under him), I hoped that if he caught me again he might do the decent thing and take a detour. He didn't! Exactly the same thing happened again, and I remember shouting to him (or at least trying to!), 'Stop swimming over me!' I wasn't even competing against him! I think he did it at least once more and, by the end of the final sprint, not only was I fuming, but I was also carrying about a gallon of sea water in my stomach.

'Excuse me, Spencer,' I said, walking towards him afterwards. Actually, I was probably stomping. 'It's hard enough trying to swim 200 metres in the Pacific Ocean with waves crashing around without being submerged by a giant every five minutes!'

These blokes are an absolute nightmare.

Going back to my first triathlon, it wasn't actually the swim that caused me the biggest problem, it was the wetsuit. After deciding to take part in this triathlon, which was taking place in Yorkshire somewhere, I had gone out and bought myself my first ever wetsuit.

'Make sure you practise getting in and out of it,' recommended one of the boys at work. 'Otherwise you could be in big trouble.'

Having never competed in or even seen a triathlon before, I had no idea that what he really meant was, make sure you practise getting out of your wetsuit in a hurry. As I was soon to find out, the difference between removing a wetsuit quickly and removing one in a leisurely way is significant and it's one of those memories that when I repeat it in my head it's always in slow motion. After completing the swim, which I didn't enjoy one bit, I made my way to the transition area and as everyone else started tearing their wetsuits off at a hundred miles an hour I started doing the same. I got it as far as my ankles but when I started trying to remove it completely I realised that it had bunched up. And I mean *properly* bunched up.

I can't repeat what I started saying under my breath but as my fellow triathletes came and went I spent about seven minutes hopping around the transition area, falling on my front and my backside and swearing like a trooper. It must have been a pathetic sight. Seven minutes, though. That's appalling.

As much as I enjoyed improving my swimming, and I genuinely did enjoy it, there were times when I longed to run and cycle but not swim. It's no surprise then that after a while I started competing in duathlons too. From a pleasure point of view these were heaven for me, and it wasn't long before I was competing at quite a high level. In fact, my last competitive race before taking up CrossFit full time was at the 2010 Duathlon World Championships in Edinburgh – more on that later.

Despite the swimming, I still enjoyed signing up for triathlons from time to time and when I competed they produced some of my best performances. Not necessarily in all three events, it has to be said, but at least one usually went well. One that springs to mind is the Leeds Triathlon that took place in Roundhay Park in 2008 or 2009. It was freezing cold for the swim and somewhere along the way I encountered a dead goose floating in the water, which was nice! I got cramp soon after that and with nothing to grab onto (we were in the middle of a big lake) I had to complete at least half of the swim without the use of one leg and in extreme pain. When I finally extracted myself from the lake I was really fed up and because I was also a bit disorientated I couldn't find my bike. I managed to get my wetsuit off, though, which was a bonus! After eventually tracking down the bike, I set off, and after a few minutes I started to get my second wind. Actually, this was my first wind really as until now I hadn't really been at the races.

I have no idea where I was placed when I started the run but by that time I was definitely back in contention. With nothing to lose and with plenty of energy still left in the tank I decided to floor it, and I ended up finishing fourth overall. I forget the time, but I ran my fastest ever 10k. If it hadn't been for cramp and that poor dead goose, who knows?

Before I tell you about how I got into CrossFit I should mention that, despite all my endeavours in sport, in 2009, which is when I started to become interested in CrossFit, I was nothing more than a good all-rounder. Although I may have had promise as an athlete, I hadn't done anything that could have been considered to be outstanding. I'd been part of the Bradford City ladies' team when they'd won the County Cup and I'd also carried my bike across the finish line having crashed it during a race, but until sometime after I became involved in CrossFit I had no ambitions whatsoever to become a full-time athlete.

Nor did I think I had it in me, to be honest. I was determined (ridiculously so, some would say), had good stamina, was fairly strong and I could hold my own in most of the sports I practised. The fittest on earth though? I was a firefighter at the end of the day. A firefighter who was into sport. It was as simple as that.

I was also approaching my late twenties, which is when some athletes and sportspeople are at their peak or are even starting to slow down. People often assume that prior to taking up CrossFit I'd been winning triathlons left, right and centre and had been a kind of world beater in training. If only! What's perhaps more interesting is that, despite me competing in triathlons and duathlons, I'd played team sports mainly, which I touched on earlier. Even at the running club I excelled in events like the cross-country relay and the road relays, so I was a team player first and foremost. That was definitely my forte. The social side still played a big part so back then the thought of being on my own in a sport would have felt a bit unnatural.

What started shifting my mentality a bit were my performances in triathlons and duathlons. In duathlons I managed to qualify for the world championships and in the triathlons the European championships, so they were probably the first signs of me being happier competing as an individual. Either way, I was just enjoying myself and the last thing I was expecting was to become obsessed by a sport that would ultimately take over the lot.

CHAPTER 10:

A PERFECT FIT

As you'll have already gathered, the fire stations I was based at were full of people who took their fitness quite seriously. As well as all the cycling, football and triathlons I've mentioned, we also used to lift weights together and that's another thing that the boys used to encourage me with. There were always men's fitness magazines lying around at the station and more often than not there'd be a power workout in them which we'd always end up doing. Looking back, these workouts were usually quite CrossFit-esque and on my days off I'd go to my gym and do something similar. One day, shortly after completing one of these workouts, I was approached by one of the personal trainers at the gym who suggested I try CrossFit.

'I've been watching you train,' he said, 'and I think CrossFit would suit you.'

'Cross what?' I replied. I'd honestly never heard of it.

The trainer, who had offered to take me to a class if I liked the look of it, very kindly wrote it down on a piece of paper and when I got home I Googled it. The website I found said something along the lines of: 'CrossFit is both a physical exercise philosophy and a competitive fitness sport, incorporating elements from high-intensity interval training, weightlifting, plyometrics, powerlifting, gymnastics, strongman, and other exercises.' As somebody who likes a bit of variety with their sport this was right up my street, so, after doing a bit more research, I went back in the next day and told him I'd like to give it a go.

Believe it or not, apart from the sport's physical diversity, the reason I decided to try it was because it sounded quite sociable. As a firefighter I'd work two days and two nights before having four days off, which were usually during the week. Because the majority of people I knew would always be working during this time, I needed something to occupy me. If I wasn't doing something physical that just left housework.

Me and housework have always had quite a strange relationship, incidentally. Things have changed slightly since my teens. After my mum would force me to tidy up my bedroom, I'd aim to keep it tidy but would always find an excuse not to do so. Then, when it's just this side of dangerous – i.e. there's several weeks' worth of washing that needs putting away and I can barely see the carpet – I'll force myself to blitz it and it'll start all over again.

Anyway, this need to escape the housework combined with my usual desire to try new things made me think I should definitely give CrossFit a shot. My first ever CrossFit class took place at a gym called CrossFit Central Manchester and the person taking the class was the owner and head coach there, Simon Jones. The venue itself was a unit on an industrial estate and it was cold and very basic – a world away from Virgin Active where I was a member. When I first walked in I remember thinking, *Wow, this is a bit weird*. It was a bit like turning up to a new class like you'd do at a gym, except I literally had no idea what I was going to be doing. I'd obviously been given the lowdown about what CrossFit entailed, but it was all very general.

What helped to relax me a bit were the people. At Virgin Active it was always a bit of a lottery as to what the atmosphere would be like – partly because the people were usually training alone but it was also down to what kind of mood people were in. Sometimes the atmosphere would be warm and friendly and sometimes it wouldn't. This was a completely different kettle of fish and everyone was super-friendly. All of a sudden the venue, which I'd initially found unwelcoming, didn't matter any more.

I can't remember what skill we did that day but the workout was called 'Helen', which is three rounds of a 400-metre run, twenty-one kettlebell swings and twelve pull-ups. I was a good runner and could already do strict pull-ups so I was able to do the workout and push hard. I remember thinking afterwards that it was all pretty cool and that I could see myself doing this every day. By the time I got home I'd made the decision to do so, and the following day I cancelled my membership with Virgin Active. The rest, as they say, is history!

I still had commitments to other sporting activities, of course, though all the other disciplines fed into my general fitness, which helped with CrossFit and vice versa. At the time of my first CrossFit class I was training for a triathlon and running for my club, and the person taking the class said that, as well as helping to improve my times in both of these, CrossFit would also improve my overall strength and stamina. Four for the price of one, basically.

He was right. After just a few weeks of doing CrossFit, my times in both the triathlons and running had improved massively and I was well and truly hooked. It ticked every single box for me, physically and socially, and the more I went the more interested I became in its development and ethos. I'm assuming that the majority of people reading this book will have practised CrossFit, or will at least have a knowledge of it or interest in it. If my assumption is correct you'll know just how all-encompassing CrossFit can be and how it can turn your life upside down. In a good way. Personally, it felt like I'd finally found something that matched my character, personality and outlook on life. Something varied and community-driven that required discipline, commitment and a whole lot of effort. CrossFit could almost have been made for me, and me for CrossFit.

One of my first spinoffs from doing CrossFit, as in something my trainer recommended I try that might benefit me on my CrossFit journey, was indoor rowing and, in November 2009, some boys from the gym and I entered the British Indoor Rowing Championships. This became yet another mini-adventure for me and I ended up becoming the British lightweight champion. What brought me back down to earth was that shortly after my row one of the officials came up to see me (I was dying on the floor at the time) and said, and I quote, 'That was some of the worst technique I have ever seen by a rowing champion. But congratulations on the win, of course.' I didn't know whether to hug him or punch him!

About a month after competing at the indoor rowing championship, I was asked if I'd be interested in entering a CrossFit competition and naturally I said yes. Yes please, in fact. The sport was still very much in its infancy, certainly in this country, but the people who were doing CrossFit were already dedicated and the standard was getting higher all the time. The number of girls who'd entered this competition was quite small – about ten, I think – so the organisers decided the men and women should do the trail run together. It was a 5k run and I ended up beating everybody, including the boys. As well as beating everyone in the trail run, I also beat the other girls overall, so all things considered it wasn't a bad start to my CrossFit career. In fact, it was an excellent start.

I went into the end of 2009 on a bit of a high really. Manchester now felt like home and things at work couldn't have been better. Mourning the loss of football had lasted a matter of days and, thanks to running, rowing, the triathlons and duathlons and especially CrossFit, my fitness and social life had been improving almost daily. Finishing off the year with a win at my maiden CrossFit competition had been the icing on the Christmas cake and the only downer was that I had no idea when the next competition would be.

Fortunately, due to me being rushed off my feet with life in general, I didn't have time to let this bother me. Then, in February 2010, somebody at my gym suggested that I enter the UK and Ireland Sectional competition. Sectionals were precursors to the CrossFit Open and, because CrossFit was still in its infancy over here, the UK and Ireland had been grouped together. To put this into perspective with regards to how far in front the USA were at the time, California had its own Sectional. That said, because you had to finish in the top three in order to progress to the Regionals, I'm glad I was competing over here and not over there as I have a feeling the competition might have been a bit stiffer.

Because I'd only competed in one CrossFit competition, I was unsure about entering the Sectional but the people at the gym wouldn't take no for an answer.

'Come on,' they said. 'It'll be a laugh. We'll hire a minibus, book a hotel and we'll all go down together.'

Put like that, it did sound quite attractive.

'Go on then,' I said. 'Let's give it a go.'

For all my determination and endeavour I was still finding my feet with CrossFit and I didn't want to get too ahead of myself after winning just one competition. Then again, the ethos behind CrossFit is long-term health for every individual so by competing in another competition, regardless of its importance, I was merely upholding that philosophy. The only potential issue I had was work. I was due on that weekend and this wasn't the first time I'd had to ask to swap shifts with somebody. I had a feeling that it was going to become a regular thing.

It was meant to be held at Mildenhall air base in Suffolk, but, due to complications with getting on to the base, it was moved to Jubilee Fields in the centre of Mildenhall. The weather was absolutely atrocious (what, in the UK in March?) and, after having moved the events from being indoors to outdoors right at the last minute, it was touch and go as to whether it would all go ahead. Fortunately, after a huge canopy was erected, the events took place without a hitch and I managed to win all three – the CTB/GHD/wall ball, DU/GTOH/TTB and Row/Load/Run – quite convincingly. For the uninitiated, this stands for chest-to-bar pull-ups (CTB); sit-ups on a glute-ham developer machine (GHD); squatting and throwing a heavy ball against a wall in an explosive movement (wall ball); double-under jumps with a skipping rope (DU); lifting a plate or bar from ground to overhead (GTOH); and a toes-to-bar gymnastic movement that is done hanging from a bar (TTB). We like our acronyms in CrossFit!

The upshot of me winning the UK and Ireland Sectional was that I'd qualified for the European Regional, but my excitement was tempered slightly by the fact that I'd have to ask for more time off work. Luckily, I shouldn't have had any worries at all in that department as everybody at my station was just pleased and proud that I'd progressed and it wasn't a case of finding somebody to help, it was a case of choosing which person.

With everything at work sorted, I was able to concentrate on the European Regional, which was taking place in May. My expectations for this event were low and I promise you that's not false modesty. I'd been told, quite rightly, that this was going to be on a very different scale to the Sectional or the first event, certainly in terms of competition. It was a step into the unknown.

As with the Sectional, we had a minibus-full for the Regional competition and among its six passengers, who were all from my gym, was another competitor and somebody who was going to be judging. My attitude going into this competition was actually more relaxed than the Sectional, as I had no ambitions other than to have fun and enjoy myself. We were all in the same boat in that respect and when we set off I was really excited.

The venue for the competition was in a remote part of Sweden and after arriving at our hotel quite late we dumped our stuff in our rooms and headed out for something to eat. This is where the remoteness of the venue started to have an effect as the waitress in the restaurant we went to didn't speak a single word of English. Unfortunately, our Swedish, which we'd learned from watching the chef on *The Muppet Show*, was even worse so we were in danger of starving. After about ten minutes, during which time the waitress had gone to great lengths trying to explain what we could have to eat, we settled on something described as a Bambi Burger that we think was a venison burger. It could have been whale for all I know. Ordering the lager was an awful lot easier – four fingers and the word Carlsberg did it – so, on the night before a competition that would potentially catapult me into the CrossFit Games, I was drinking beer and eating burgers with some friends! My preparation has changed a bit since then. These days I drink slightly less beer and I definitely wouldn't do so one day before a competition!

Once again, the weather played its part in the proceedings, except this time we were moved from outdoors to indoors. It didn't affect the events though. The athlete who came with the biggest reputation was Iceland's Annie Thorisdottir who has become a really good friend of mine and is obviously an immense athlete. In 2009, she'd finished eleventh at the CrossFit Games and was the first non-American to do well. Instead of being intimidated by competing against someone of her standard, I was really looking forward to it. She was the benchmark, at least in our region, and I wanted to be tested.

On the first day Annie and I won one event each: she won the overhead carry and I won the run. This was obviously a shot in the arm to me as I hadn't been expecting to win anything. In fact, the only thing guaranteed after the first day was that the competition was fierce and nobody, not even Annie, who I should point out is over seven years younger than I am, could take their spot for granted. At the start of day two, Annie pulled away slightly, which left me, Jenny Magnusdottir and Ingunn Oftedal all fighting for the remaining two places. By winning the final, which I did by 22 seconds, I secured second place on the podium and a place at the 2010 CrossFit Games, which were being held in Los Angeles. I couldn't believe it.

Keeping my expectations low had been sensible but then elevating them when I realised I had a chance had been just as important. It's all very well adapting to situations physically, but if you can't do it mentally, especially at this level, then you're going to be in big trouble. To be honest I didn't have to do very much as the excitement of being able to hold my own against the likes of

Annie and potentially qualify for the CrossFit Games was enough to get me through. It still had to be managed, though. Everything has to be managed. And this time, it seemed that both my mental and physical preparation had definitely paid off. I was now on my way to the 2010 CrossFit Games, the biggest sporting event of my life so far.

CHAPTER 11:

ENTER THE ENGINE

Back in Manchester, the enormity of what I'd just achieved was starting to sink in. In less than two months' time I would be flying out to California to compete at the 2010 CrossFit Games. Or would I? First I had to sort out my work schedule and with no time off left to play with I'd have to go cap in hand once again and start asking to swap shifts. At the risk of repeating myself, the boys at the station were just fantastic and yet again they bent over backwards to help. The job still came first. That was never in question. I was doing something different though, and as well as everyone taking an interest it seemed to be good for morale.

The thought of going to Los Angeles, let alone competing at the CrossFit Games, was quite a big deal for me. I'd only been to America once as part of a school ski trip, where obviously everything was organised and planned for us! My usual trips never went further than the Greek islands! I'd only ventured to London once or twice. It was going to be a real adventure.

Something else I hadn't done prior to qualifying for the 2010 CrossFit Games was acquire any sponsors. Selling myself commercially has never been one of my strong points and, although I've always been quite a gregarious person, the thought of going up to somebody and asking them for money or support in return for me wearing some logos filled me with dread. To be honest, it still does. I mean, what on earth do you say? On the few occasions I've tried to do it I've always ended up either getting tongue-tied or sounding like a character from a Dickens novel. Please, sir, could I have some money please? Fortunately for me, my stepdad, Andy, offered to help me out and he managed to persuade a training equipment manufacturer called Beaver Fit to pay for me to fly out there. In return I had to wear a T-shirt with their logo on the front while I was competing. When the T-shirts arrived a couple of days before I left for LA I realised that as well as being quite large they were made out of very thick fabric. Exactly what I needed in the California sunshine!

On Tuesday, 13 July, after work I got packed and on the Wednesday I flew out to Los Angeles with my then partner who was accompanying me. The next day I had to check in at the venue and on the Friday night I started competing. Talk about cutting it fine! Ideally now athletes like to go out there at least two or three weeks beforehand just to acclimatise and get used to the time difference. But there was no time for things like jetlag in this instance. It was literally jump off the plane, dump your stuff, register and compete. Sam Briggs' four steps to competing in the CrossFit Games, 2010-style!

It's hard to put into words the difference between the Regionals back then and the Games. At the Regionals, which had taken place in a gym and a parking lot, there'd been maybe a hundred people there and at least half of them had been competitors. It was a great atmosphere, but the majority of that atmosphere had been generated by the competitors themselves. So when I arrived in LA I still hadn't competed in front of a large crowd – not in CrossFit, at least. Overall I think the largest crowd I'd ever competed in front of at this point was at Odsal Top with the school rugby team. The difference being that we were just a sideshow that day and nobody there had come to see two girls' teams compete.

This, then, was a completely new experience. The capacity of the StubHub Center, which is in Carson City, California, is about 27,000 and on the Friday night it must have been at least two-thirds full. Because the sport was created in America, the following CrossFit had, and the reaction from the fans, was completely different to the UK and Sweden. They also had no problem showing their emotions and the noise they created, especially for the final, was just incredible. The other big difference was that I obviously had no team behind me. It was just me, myself and I. That in itself was actually quite invigorating and instead of feeling intimidated by it I felt galvanised. Perhaps it was fight or flight kicking in? I could either let it all affect me and collapse into an emotional heap or I could grasp the nettle and give it everything I had. The former was never going to happen.

The first event of the 2010 CrossFit Games was 'Amanda', which is one of the classic CrossFit workouts named after a competitor called Amanda Miller who tragically succumbed to cancer a year after she had competed in an American Regional. It featured, for time, 9-7-5 reps of squat snatches at my current 1-rep max paired with muscle-ups. I managed to get through the nines and sevens okay but that was as far as I got and I ended up finishing twentieth out of forty-three competitors. Fast forward to the 2017 CrossFit Games and I managed forty-five reps in a similar event and finished third. How times have changed. I suppose I could try to blame jetlag or a lack of preparation for that finish but the truth is that's where I deserved to be. I was still a relative beginner, so a top-half finish wasn't that bad.

The next event was the 'Pyramid Double Helen' (many CrossFit workouts are given names), which consisted of a 1,200-metre run,

63 kettlebell swings, 36 pull-ups, an 800-metre run, 42 kettlebell swings, 24 pull-ups, a 400-metre run, 21 kettlebell swings and 12 pull-ups – all to be completed within a 22-minute time limit. After my heat, Miranda Oldroyd interviewed me and told me the commentator had said I'd gone out too hard and would never be able to sustain the pace. He obviously had no idea that I'd been running for a club and had been competing in duathlons and triathlons for a few years! She made the point I obviously had a good engine, and this comment was repeated several times after other endurance events over the years, until eventually people started to call me 'the Engine'. As nicknames go it's quite a good one so I'm happy it stuck.

I won my heat in the Pyramid Double Helen and came third overall in that event, though I didn't find out until after the final heat. It ended up being my best event of the Games; everything after that was mid-table. But the reaction I received for finishing third in the Helen was amazing. Nobody there had ever heard of me, yet when my name was called out everybody seemed to go crazy.

'In third place, from the UK, Sam Briggs!'

'YAAAAAAAAAAAAAAAAY!'

Really? Thanks!

I'm not going to pretend that didn't feel fantastic, because it did. It also opened my ears to the crowd a bit more and from then on I was able to tap into the energy they created. There's no booing in CrossFit. People obviously have their favourites but at the end of the day everyone wants everyone to do well.

In order to qualify for the final event you had to be in the top ten after the penultimate event, and unfortunately I only managed nineteenth. But I was more than happy with that – as it was my first year of doing CrossFit, I had come with no expectations so finishing nineteenth seemed pretty good to me. But I remember sitting in the stands afterwards with a large beer in my hand thinking, *Next year I want to be in the final.* That might have been the beer talking but when I left the stadium that night I'd already forgotten about what I'd achieved since starting CrossFit. It was what I was *going* to achieve that mattered. I was fully motivated and just wanted to see how far I could go within the sport.

I'm afraid I don't remember this as well as Mum does, but at my first CrossFit Games Mum remembers watching me in a run and pull-up event where my strength and enthusiasm were undone by my lack of experience. Mum wasn't able to be there in person so was watching it online and apparently in the run I was lapping the other girls with ease and making mincemeat of them. When it came to the pull-ups, however, they were all doing the butterfly variety, whereas I was doing them the old-fashioned way. Consequently, what should have been a walk in the park to first place for me ended up being a loss. I'm told that the watching Americans were all flabbergasted by my performance. I was quite a bit smaller than everyone else, so nobody had taken much notice of me. Then all of sudden, BOOM! Out of the blocks I went. Although I didn't win the event, I certainly made an impression.

The best thing about appearing at the CrossFit Games in 2010 was that it helped me appreciate where I stood in terms of how good I was and how good I needed to be. Collectively, the Americans were still light years away from everyone else but coming third in the Helen had made me realise that they weren't unbeatable and that if I kept on working hard I could definitely make the final next year. That was my goal and when I arrived back in England I was raring to go.

When I arrived back at work, my boss asked me if I'd like to become the station fitness instructor and you won't be surprised to learn that I bit his hand off. I'd have to take some exams, of course, but that didn't matter. I thought it was an absolutely fabulous idea and, from a personal point of view, it was obviously ideal. When I finally took up the post I suggested to the boys that we integrate CrossFit into the training and they were all enthusiastic. One of them used to be a carpenter so he made us some boxes and we also put some rings up. Being able to practise CrossFit during working hours, albeit sometimes interrupted by call-outs, brought me even closer to the sport, and the fact that the boys all took an interest and seemed to enjoy it was amazing. I now had CrossFit and the fire service running in tandem. It was the perfect situation really.

The other big decision to come from that trip was my retirement from competing in duathlons and triathlons. I knew I was fit enough to compete in CrossFit, but my strength was lacking, and all the endurance training for the triathlons meant it was hard to gain strength. I wanted to focus my efforts on CrossFit to see if I could get into that top ten and make the final in 2011.

However, when I made the decision, I was already through to the Duathlon World Championships in Edinburgh so I wanted to see how I could fare in that. Let's face it, getting to wear a GB suit with my surname on was pretty cool, plus I'd already bought an expensive race bike when I'd qualified for the occasion! Oh, and me being me, there were just a *couple* of other things I needed to get out of my system when it came to other sports too . . .

CHAPTER 12:

DING DING, SECONDS OUT ...

Two months after the CrossFit Games, I went up to Edinburgh to compete in the World Duathlon Championships. With CrossFit now taking up nearly all of my time I didn't really train as much as I'd have liked and I ended up finishing eighth in my age group. It was quite a big field so that wasn't a bad result but the fact is my heart wasn't in it any more. Incidentally, I was asked once if I'd ever fancied competing in a biathlon and until recently it was something I was keen to have a go at. Then, at the Rogue Invitational this year, I had a go with a gun and it appears that I might not be suited to the event. Actually, that's an understatement. The American and Scandinavian athletes were all fantastic but I was just a liability. Nobody got hurt, fortunately, and at least it means I'll never have to go cross-country skiing.

Something else I had a go at in 2010 was white-collar boxing. Yes, I thought that might come as a surprise. It happened through the fire service, and when the idea was first suggested to me my initial thought was: *What will Mum say?* Once I'd put that to bed I thought, *Yes, why not?* It was all part of a big charity event and the bouts on the card were all Leeds District firefighters versus Bradford District firefighters. We each had to have six months' training for the fights so they took it very seriously. So did we, to be honest, and if CrossFit hadn't been so prevalent in my life it's something I might have done more frequently.

The only issue I had prior to the bout was my weight. The girl I was due to fight, Sarah Dunn, weighed about 69 kilos and I only weighed about 61 kilos. Apparently we wouldn't be allowed to fight with that much of a difference, so the only option was for her to try to lose and me to put some weight on. Fortunately, I quite like eating so that wasn't a problem and the man who was training me gave me some tips as to what to eat. About a week before the fight I was still slightly under my target so he ordered me to have a couple of beers every night. 'No problem whatsoever,' I said.

When I weighed in I was exactly 65 kilos and in order for me to be able to fight I had to be at least ... 65 kilos. Thank goodness for those beers!

Despite it being for charity, I was definitely going for a knockout and I was surprised at how pumped I felt beforehand. Then again, six months is a long time to train for something that might only last a few minutes, and there are no two ways about it, I wanted to win. In addition to the fact I had done contact sports as a child such as karate and kickboxing, I'd also grown up surrounded by boys. Obviously I had my brother, but my cousins were all boys too, as were the kids next door to my grandparents. From as early as I can remember I'd had to be able to look after myself and, although that ability had been dormant for a while, it was now well and truly awake again.

Because she was a bigger athlete than me, I knew my opponent would be a little slower and tire quicker, but would have more power behind her punch. The last thing I wanted to do was to give her an opportunity to put her weight advantage to use. This meant I had to come out of the blocks quite sharply while also biding my time, and my game plan until the final round was basically to try to tire Sarah out. She did manage to land a couple of punches but by the final round she was tiring, and so with the clock ticking down I decided to take my chance. I managed to land a really good upper cut and Sarah hadn't been expecting it. After falling backwards, she hit the canvas with a thud. As the referee started his count, I remember thinking, *Wow, this is like a real boxing match!*

I forget how far he got but with a few seconds to go Sarah managed to drag herself up and a few seconds after that the final bell went. While not getting my knockout, I was sure I'd done enough to get a unanimous win. Isn't that what they say in boxing? When the referee called the bout a tie my mouthguard almost fell out but I obviously didn't say anything. You'll have to forgive me for sounding competitive but that's what boxing does to you. I'm pretty sure she felt the same. More importantly, a lot of money was raised for charity that night, and after putting in a good shift I managed to lose some of my beer belly.

Speaking of which ...

The British Indoor Rowing Championships were due to take place on the Sunday after the bout, which was on a Thursday. In order to compete as a lightweight and defend my title from the previous year, I had to be under 61.5 kilos, which meant losing over 3.5 kilos in just three days. Had I had nothing else to do that would have been quite easy, I suppose, as I could have done some exercise and then sat in a sauna all day. But as well as having to work in between the bout and the championships I was also having to train, and in order to be able to train – and work – I had to eat.

The beer, incidentally, had been a deliberate decision. As the calories are empty, the resulting beer bloat should be easier to get rid of. That had been the idea. It still wasn't going to be easy, though, and in a desperate attempt to lose at least the required amount I ended up on my exercise bike in front of the fire for ninety minutes after work every night with at least five layers of clothing on. The only upside was that I was able to watch television while doing it but the task itself was pretty dire. I did this for the two nights before the row and in addition to becoming an expert in several soap operas I managed to get my weight down to exactly 61.5 kilos.

I cannot tell you the relief I felt when I found out I'd done it, but I vowed there and then never to do it again. Cutting weight is horrendous! Saying that, I wouldn't bet against me taking part in another boxing match one day, providing it was for charity. For a start, I really enjoyed the training and as a sport it seems to suit me. Some of the boys at work tried persuading me to do MMA after the bout and, although I was definitely interested, the answer had to be no. Unless I can commit to something fully, I won't – sorry, can't – get involved. There's just no point. It's all or nothing with me. At that point my mind was clear I wanted to concentrate on CrossFit, so I couldn't commit the time to other sports. And now I'd got these other things out of my system, I could concentrate on what was really important to me: qualifying for the 2011 CrossFit Games.

For 2011, the powers that be at CrossFit decided to ditch the Sectionals in favour of a mass-participation event taking place at gyms throughout the world entitled the Open. The CrossFit website describes the Open as: 'where grassroots meets greatness

– compete with hundreds of thousands of athletes in CrossFit's largest all-inclusive event'. That's it in a nutshell really. After you sign up online, the people at CrossFit release one workout each week over five to six weeks. You then do those workouts at your gym where they're filmed and then submitted to CrossFit HQ, where the numbers are crunched and the performances ranked.

In terms of community this has been tremendous, as it literally brings everyone together, regardless of ability or age. Everyone who wants to take part, that is. Even those CrossFitters who don't take part will feel engaged, as the chances are they'll be encouraging people at their gyms who are competing, so everyone plays a part. It must be one of the most inclusive competitions in world sport and is the essence of CrossFit.

As 2011 was my first ever Open, I'm going to list all six of the workouts:

Week 1
Complete as many rounds and reps as possible in 10 minutes of:
30 double-unders
15 power snatches (55lb/25kg)

Week 2
Complete as many rounds and reps as possible in 15 minutes of:
9 deadlifts (100lb/45kg)
12 push-ups
15 box jumps (20 inches/50cm high)

Week 3
Complete as many rounds and reps as possible in 5 minutes of:
Squat clean and jerk (110lb/50kg)

Week 4
Complete as many rounds and reps as possible in 10 minutes of:
60 bar-facing burpees
30 overhead squats (90lb/40kg) – a deep squat holding a bar above the head
10 muscle-ups – transitioning from hanging from some rings to a supported position, arms straight, above them

Week 5
Complete as many rounds and reps as possible in 20 minutes of:
5 power cleans (100lb/45kg)
10 toes-to-bar
15 wall balls (14lb/6kg to a 9-inch/23cm target)

Week 6
Complete as many reps as possible in 7 minutes following the rep scheme below:
65lb/30kg thruster, 3 reps (a thruster is a combination of a front squat and overhead press)
3 chest-to-bar pull-ups
65lb/30kg thruster, 6 reps
6 chest-to-bar pull-ups

65lb/30kg thruster, 9 reps

9 chest-to-bar pull-ups . . . [etc.]

Keep increasing the number of thrusters/pull-ups by three each round until the time runs out.

One of the best things about the Open is that it lets everyone who takes part know not only where they stand in the world, which is actually quite fun when you think about it, but also where you stand in your region. This was obviously of greater interest to me as it would determine my passage to the Regionals and, ultimately, the Games. In the end the barometer for where I stood in my region matched where I potentially stood in the world as the two people who beat me in the 2011 CrossFit Open were the two athletes who'd taken first and second place at the 2010 CrossFit Games: Kristan Clever and Annie Thorisdottir. It's obviously not an exact science but standing on the podium with those two (okay, it was a virtual podium) was hugely encouraging and I knew that the two months leading up to the Regionals were going to be pivotal.

The stock-in-trade piece of advice I was offered around this time by people at the gym and the boys at work was simple: keep on doing what you've been doing. It sounds simplistic but that was exactly right. I'd been making steady but excellent progress and providing I carried on I'd have a good chance at getting through to the Games again. Before that I obviously had the Regionals to contend with, which this year were being held at the Bolton Arena so a lot closer to home. The whole event was especially poignant for me as it was the first and last time my grandad, who was really unwell at the time, was able to watch me compete at CrossFit before he died, so for him to be there cheering me on was just amazing. As a young man he'd been quite a good weightlifter so for the lifting events we were able to get him to the front of the stands so he could see the action close up. You'll never, ever see me give anything less than 100 per cent but with Grandad there my will to succeed was even greater than usual.

The first event at the 2011 European Regional was a 1k run followed by thirty handstand push-ups against a wall (yes, they are exactly as fiendish as they sound) and a 1k row. There was a 15-minute time cap; if you went over the time, a 1-second penalty was added for each metre not covered or each handstand not completed.

The next event was a thruster ladder in which we had 20 seconds to take a barbell from the ground and then perform one thruster at a specified weight. We then had 20 seconds to transition to the next – slightly heavier – barbell where the same thing applied. We were only allowed to make one thruster attempt in any 20-second period, by the way, so if you fluffed one you were out, no second chances. There were fifteen barbells in all and we obviously had to get to the highest weight possible. If an athlete wasn't able to complete a successful thruster with the first barbell, they received a DNF ('did not finish') and were eliminated from the competition.

Event three was 21-15-9 reps for time of deadlifts and then box jumps ('for time' just means the workout is timed so you are ranked on how quickly you can complete it). Event four was, again for time, 100 pull-ups, 100 kettlebell swings, 100 double-unders and 100 overhead squats. Event five, 'Amanda', was 9-7-5 reps for time of muscle-ups and squat snatches (a repeat of the first workout I'd done at the Games) and event six was, for time, row 20 calories (in other words, for as long as it takes to burn off 20 calories according to the rowing machine), thirty burpees, forty two-arm dumbbell ground-to-overheads, fifty toes-to-bar, 100-foot/30m overhead walking lunges carrying a 25lb/11kg plate and, last but not least, a 150-foot/45m sprint.

As well as it taking place on home soil, there appeared to be a lot more interest in this year's competition and, instead of all the outdoor events taking place in a car park like they had done in 2010, they were staged within an athletic stadium. Subsequently, the whole thing felt a lot more professional. Something else I noticed this year that I hadn't noticed previously was the crowd. As well as being a lot bigger, there were more English voices present among the Europeans. What I found funny was trying to pick out the English cheers amongst the other languages.

In the first event, Annie beat my time by about 20 seconds and in event two she did a 175lb/79kg thruster to my 155lb/70kg. Event three went the same way, as did event four, but with event five, Amanda, I managed to get one over on her by posting a time of 9:56 to her 11:49. For the last event we swapped times almost, which gave Annie five events to my one. At the time, Annie wasn't just the best female CrossFit athlete in Europe, but potentially in the world, so finishing second to her at the 2011 European Regional was an incredible achievement and I took nothing from it but encouragement and pride.

As well as hard work, the changes I'd made since last year had paid dividends, not least my change in diet. I'm not saying I used to eat burgers every day – and in any case, the changes I made weren't wholesale. It was more a case of refining my diet, really. Things like beer, for instance, although enjoyable, simply wasn't conducive to me succeeding as an athlete so it had to become an occasional treat. That was definitely one of my weaknesses.

I once read an interview with a strength athlete called Eddie Hall who, in 2016, managed to deadlift 500kg. In the six months leading up to the deadlift he was eating about 13,000 calories a day and about two hours before the lift he went into a restaurant for his final meal.

'Do you happen to have a large gammon joint?' Eddie asked the waiter.

'Yes sir, we do,' he replied.

'Well, could you take the fat off for me please and bring it to me on a plate?'

'What, bring the gammon to you on a plate?' asked the waiter.

'No,' said Eddie. 'I want the fat!'

How horrid is that? Luckily, I didn't have to go to such extremes when it came to my own eating regime.

What really helped me diet-wise at the time was something called the Zone Diet, which is used widely in CrossFit. It's all about portioning your meals correctly and it encourages a balance of lean proteins, non-starchy vegetables, nuts, seeds and low-glycaemic fruit, while limiting starch and refined sugar. I was definitely a little bit late to this side of things (there's a pattern growing here!) but once I got into it I became really interested and I still am. Prior to taking up CrossFit, my daily eating patterns had been all over the place and a typical training day might start with a big bowl of cereal in the morning, followed by a run and then another bowl of cereal. After that I'd go to the gym and at some point during the afternoon I'd have some pasta or a sandwich, and perhaps a snack. The point being that a source of protein wouldn't usually touch my lips until after I'd finished training, which is obviously ridiculous. A good diet, at whatever level you train, is absolutely essential; not just to your fitness but to your general health and wellbeing. As somebody who found this out the hard way, I cannot stress this enough.

With my diet revamped and my place in the 2011 CrossFit Games assured, I could look forward to what lay ahead with confidence. Was 2011 going to be my year?

CHAPTER 13:

WHAT'S A SOFTBALL?

The biggest difference for me between the CrossFit Games 2010 and the CrossFit Games 2011 was preparation. No need for me to change shifts at work this year: I'd already booked a two-week holiday. And instead of just two of us going, there were going to be six or seven, and my parents would be making the trip too. Team Briggs, as we were, consisted of me, my partner and some friends of ours, and after the Games were over we were all going to travel up to Yosemite for a few days and then across to San Francisco. It was a holiday, basically, with a rather important sporting competition in the middle. Having a group of friends in the audience was going to be special, as was having a Union Jack or two being waved. I couldn't wait to get over there.

The element of surprise is obviously an important facet of CrossFit. As I've already said, you have to be ready for absolutely anything and over the years the organisers of the Games have sprung some absolute whoppers on us. I'm not going to do this for every competition, but to demonstrate just how mad and eclectic this can get, I'm going to list the first six events from the 2011 CrossFit Games.

Event 1 – Beach

For time:

210-metre ocean swim

1,500-metre soft-sand run

50 chest-to-bar pull-ups

100 hand-release push-ups

200 squats

1,500-metre soft-sand run

Event 2 – Dog Sled

Three rounds for time of:

30 double-unders

95lb/43kg overhead squats, 10 reps

Then three rounds of:

10 handstand push-ups

40-foot/12-metre sled push (pushing a sled + 275lb/125kg load)

Event 3 – Killer Kage

Three rounds for time of:

155lb/70kg front squats, 7 reps

Bike 700 metres

100-foot/30-metre monkey bar traverse

Event 4 – Rope-Clean

For time:

15-foot/4.5-metre rope climb, 5 ascents

115lb/52kg clean and jerks, 5 reps

15-foot/4.5-metre rope climb, 4 ascents

125lb/57kg clean and jerks, 4 reps

15-foot/4.5-metre rope climb, 3 ascents

135lb/61kg clean and jerks, 3 reps
15-foot/4.5-metre rope climb, 2 ascents
145lb/66kg clean and jerks, 2 reps
15-foot/4.5-metre rope climb, 1 ascent
155lb/70kg clean and jerk, 1 rep

Event 5 – Skills 1
Max L-sit for time (1 attempt) – this is a gymnastic move
where you hold yourself up on some rings with your legs
extended in front of you
Max-distance softball throw (2 attempts)
Max-distance handstand walk (1 attempt with 1 mulligan
if less than 5 yards)

Event 6 – Skills 2
1-rep-max weighted chest-to-bar pull-up for load (2
minutes to complete)
1-rep-max snatch for load (2 minutes to complete)
Weighted water jug carry for distance in 60 seconds

The event that made me nervous was event number five as I'd never
even heard of softball before. Genuinely! I obviously know what it is
now, but when the organisers read out, 'Max distance softball throw,
two attempts,' my only question was: what on earth is a softball?
This was also paired with a handstand walk, which was probably my
Achilles heel, so without wanting to sound too pessimistic I didn't
fancy my chances much. In the warm-up area before the event,
Sean Lind, a gymnastics coach who I had previously met when he
was teaching a CrossFit gymnastic seminar, came up and offered to
give me some help with the handstand walk.

'Oh, yes please!' I said. 'I need all the help I can get. By the way, I don't suppose you're any good at softball, are you?'

As Sean was trying to help me, I ended up kicking him in the head by mistake. Surely this was an omen?

I managed to throw the softball over 100 feet/30 metres, as did about half the field. Then, out of the blue, up stepped Michelle Kinney who threw the ball over 190 feet/58 metres! That was an amazing effort as she's only about 5 feet 4 inches tall.

As stated in the description, the minimum distance you had to achieve in the handstand walk was five yards and that was going to be my aim. I've watched the video of this and fortunately the cameras all concentrate on the gymnasts. Then again, I was probably only on my hands for a few seconds, and when I got to the line, instead of trying to walk over it and carry on for a few more inches, I literally just threw myself in its direction and hoped for the best. It can't have been pretty. I think I achieved a distance of about 5.01 yards. If I have to be upside down, I'd rather it was on a rollercoaster!

I went into the final event, a brutal three-parter called 'The End', still tied for fifth place. Most importantly, I'd already achieved my goal for this year's CrossFit Games, which was to reach the final and so anything else from here on in would be a bonus. Incidentally, we refer to these multi-movement events as chippers and the reason for that is because you have to chip away at them. Clever, eh?

Anyway, here's what we had to do for workout number three of the last event. For time it was a 20-calorie row followed by thirty wall-ball shots with a 14lb/6kg ball, twenty toes-to-bar, thirty box jumps, twenty sumo deadlift high pulls with a 72lb/33kg kettlebell, thirty burpees, twenty shoulder-to-overheads with a

135lb/61kg barbell, and then a sled pull across the entire length of the stadium floor. This was after completing parts one and two, by the way, so by the time we went into it we'd already been on the stadium floor for about twenty minutes and in temperatures that were scorching. I'm from the UK, for heaven's sake. We don't get into the thirties there.

Although I finished the calorie row first, I was only 3 seconds in front of Annie and right behind her was Jenny LaBaw. The strongest athlete on the wall-ball shots was Rebecca Voigt, who had been one place in front of me going into the final. She was one of two athletes I had to pass on the leader board in order to make it onto the podium and so the fact that I was only a few seconds behind Rebecca motivated me to push even harder. By the fourth movement, which was the box jump, I was back in front but I was caught midway through by Julie Foucher.

The sixth movement was burpees and, having snatched the lead back from Julie, I was first to start. By the time Annie, Rebecca and Julie started the burpees I had a six-repetition advantage. That may sound like a lot, but when your body is literally screaming at you to stop and rest, six reps is nothing. Sure enough, by the time we got to the barbell, Julie had closed the gap to just three reps so there was absolutely nothing in it. Instinctively, I was trying to block out what the other girls were doing, but that was almost impossible. It's like being hunted down in a way and if the prey isn't aware of its hunter's every movement it's obviously done for. I was being hunted down by some of the fittest and most competitive women on earth and, believe me, if anything's going to make you get a shift on, or at least try to, that is!

The sled pull, which I started just 6 seconds ahead of Annie, who was now lying second in the event, isn't quite as straightforward as it sounds. Instead of simply grabbing hold of a rope and pulling a 110lb/50kg weight across a 100-foot/58-metre stadium floor, you had to run to the opposite end of the stadium, which was another 100 feet, grab hold of the heavy rope, take it back to the other end of the stadium and *then* start to pull the sled towards you. It's back-breaking! The 100 feet from the barbell to the rope felt like five times that distance and the rope itself felt like it was made from lead. I remember putting it over my shoulder and then attempting to run to the other end but the best I could manage was a very slow jog. Fortunately, everyone else seemed to be in the same situation, but when I reached the end of the stadium floor and began to pull I remember seeing Annie with a rope over her shoulder and she was literally marching with it. Iceland Annie, as she's known, was far from done and was obviously on the warpath. The crowd were going absolutely bananas and, regardless of who they were cheering for, I lapped up the energy they were creating. You can't fail to respond to an atmosphere like that. It's fantastic.

As I started to pull the sled it seemed miles away and after every exertion I just fell back in exhaustion. Annie and Julie were now well and truly on my tail and, although she was at the other end of the stadium, I could tell by the way she marched with the rope that Annie had more in the tank. It was time to call on an old friend.

With the sled now in view I decided to load it – virtually, that is – with an incentive and so from now on, instead of me staring at a sled with a weight on top of it, I was staring at a sled carrying a beautiful keg of ice-cold beer. This thing actually glistened in the sunlight and with every pull it became bigger and bigger. It sounds like a joke but it's not. I'd promised myself prior to the event that if I won I'd treat myself to a beer and so all I was doing was bringing that treat to life and making the motivation real. Or as real as my imagination could manage. It didn't let me down.

With one final heave I managed to pull the sled over the line. After doing so I stumbled to the very back of the stadium, out of the view of the cameras, and I collapsed into a heap. But this wasn't just physical exhaustion. I was mentally exhausted too, and until now that's something that had never really affected me, for the simple reason I'd never competed in such a high-profile and closely fought event.

My time in the end was 13:06, which meant that, having won the event, I had moved up to fourth position overall. I said before that anything after the final would be a bonus and finishing fourth at the 2011 CrossFit Games after winning the final event was massive. Yet another bonus, apart from the beer, which tasted absolutely incredible by the way, was the fact that the final event was also a European one/two with Annie finishing about 50 seconds behind me. She also won the title of world's fittest, so in a field that was dominated by Americans it was a big outcome and a big statement. Watch out, the Europeans are coming!

From a purely personal point of view, my improvement from last year to this had been incredible really. Not only had I kept my promise to myself but I'd put myself in a position where, if I worked just as hard again, I could get myself onto the podium and, who knows, maybe to the top step. It's strange but when I sat down and thought about my goals for 2012 I had to allow myself to get excited by the fact that perhaps I did stand a chance of becoming the fittest on earth. Had I not been capable of winning the title, I'd have been honest with myself but the fact is, I *was* capable of winning it and that in itself was extraordinarily empowering. It was a feeling that I desperately wanted to hang onto and ultimately it's what drove me forward. What also motivated me was the fact that I was far from being the finished article and had only been competing for a couple of years. The wrinkles that needed ironing out would obviously be first on my to-do list, so, although there was a lot of hard work ahead, I knew exactly what the results might bring.

Once the Games and the aftermath had come to an end, we packed up, jumped into our minibus and made our way north towards Yosemite National Park. On the second or third morning we were there, we decided to go out for a run before breakfast and we each took with us a small bottle of water. We were only going to be out for forty-five minutes, or so we thought, and we set off in the direction of some waterfalls. Three hours later we finally reached the waterfalls, which had turned out to be much further away than we'd realised, meaning we were all extremely dehydrated and hungry. In addition, one of our party twisted his ankle on the way back down. It was turning into a plot from a survival film!

Because the injured party couldn't run, we told him to make his way back down alone slowly while we raced ahead to get help. The thing is, we were so short of water by now we all needed help, not just him! Some of the boys had filled their bottles at the waterfalls, not knowing if it was safe to drink. By now we were so thirsty we were willing to try, though we had to ration it in tiny sips. Meanwhile, one of the girls in the party came across a packet of discarded jellybeans on the ground. By the way we all reacted you'd have thought she'd struck oil or found a bag of gold and after cheers and a few high fives we started rationing them out. It turned out we had enough for literally one jellybean each and that had to last us until ... actually, we had absolutely no idea! By now we were all worrying about our injured friend and regretting leaving him alone. What if he were eaten by a grizzly bear?

We finally arrived back at our lodge about seven hours after setting off and who was sitting down with his feet up having a nice little nap? That's right, Mr Twisted Ankle. He must have found a short cut and was back at the house before us.

My biggest achievement then throughout the entire two weeks wasn't busting my gut, imagining kegs of beer and finishing fourth at the 2011 CrossFit Games. It was not dying in Yosemite Park!

CHAPTER 14:

A BIT OF BAD NEWS

The late summer and early autumn of 2011 were quite quiet, CrossFit-wise, which enabled me to get used to being a firefighter again. With everything that had been going on I'd almost forgotten I had a real job, although the boys at the station did keep reminding me from time to time. The support I received from my friends, family and colleagues at this time was beyond anything I could have wished for and that support has followed me through my career. I like to think that I repay it by always doing my best but, boy, is it appreciated.

The only thing that was really niggling me after the 2011 CrossFit Games was a recurring knee problem that I'd had for a couple of years. According to the doctor, it was a maltracking of the right kneecap and had been caused by running. If you think about it, I'd been doing little else other than run since I was a child, what with football and everything. So it should have been no surprise really. More importantly, with my training now being so varied I should have had it seen to ages ago but because it was only a twinge I never bothered. It was an inconvenience more than anything. A result of wear and tear.

In November 2011, as part of my CrossFit training, I entered an Olympic weightlifting competition. While warming up I felt the usual niggle, but everything seemed as normal until the last split jerk. As I landed, I knew it was something different, but I kept trying to fight with the weight overhead, though I was unable to stand it up. I'm not saying I felt invincible, but I was still on a bit of a high after the Games and because everything had been going so well I didn't believe it could be serious. Or I didn't want to believe. Either way I wasn't listening to my body like I should have been.

You'd think that after something like this happening I'd have taken evasive action but unfortunately denial kicked in and I just carried on training. It was painful but I was used to pain so, instead of seeing a doctor and getting it sorted once and for all, I just gritted my teeth and pretended it wasn't there. The Open was just around the corner and, whether I was conscious of it or not, that was clearly a deciding factor. I'm certainly not the first athlete to ignore an injury but, if you bear in mind the level I was competing at, it was foolish beyond belief. I don't want to tell anybody what to do in this book but, if you have a niggle, please don't do what I did. Get it looked at right away.

One of the last things I did in 2011 was collect the keys to a new CrossFit gym I'd invested in with four friends. It sounds quite glamorous but I promise you it wasn't. It was basically just a big, empty, open space when we got it and the reason I got involved, apart from hopefully making some money eventually, was because Manchester didn't have many affiliate CrossFit gyms at the time and with the sport growing so quickly it seemed like a good idea. We wanted to create a space where people could come and train throughout the day, as most of the current gyms had limited classes and opening times. As someone wanting to compete, I needed more access to the gym so this seemed like the perfect solution.

The two people who were supposed to run the gym on a day-to-day basis, at least at first, were me and a friend of mine called Darren Freeman, or Daz. Daz had been a member at the gym I'd been using in Manchester and we'd become really good friends.

In fact, Daz and I had already been on one or two mini CrossFit adventures together, and one of these is worth a mention. It happened in 2010 when I was invited to attend the BodyPower Expo at the Birmingham NEC. Although growing, CrossFit was still very new in the UK at the time. Despite this, the organisers had asked me and one other athlete to do a workout demonstration on the main stage. This had meant nothing to me at the time as I'd never been to the BodyPower Expo but when Daz and I arrived at the arena with the equipment I almost died. Apparently, over the course of the event, over 80,000 people were due to visit the exhibition and you could have fitted five football teams on the main stage. It was massive!

The equipment we had was a portable pull-up rig and to be honest I don't think they were expecting someone as large as Daz to be doing pull-ups, so the rig wasn't screwed into the floor. Consequently, when Daz and I began the workout the entire rig started rocking about and we looked more like a circus act than a couple of CrossFitters. Daz was the one doing all the talking and let's just say that the audience, who were all bodybuilders, weren't impressed by either of us. In Daz's words, we died on our arses.

The kit at our new gym wasn't due to arrive until January, and when Daz and I started work on the building before then it was pretty bleak. We had to knock down walls, rip out the toilets, create changing rooms, paint the walls inside and out, lay the flooring – you name it. We had invested all our money into rent and basic equipment so all the dirty work had to be done by us and our friends as we couldn't afford to pay anyone. We had no kit, no members, no heating and, worst of all, no WiFi! Because of the time of year it was absolutely freezing so at lunchtimes we'd go back to my flat just to keep warm.

My role at the gym, apart from being an investor, was ambassadorial really and, although I was happy to help out early doors with the setup, that was only ever a temporary measure. I was a firefighter first, a CrossFitter second, and a part-owner of a gym third. The gym, which is called Train Manchester, finally opened in January 2012 and, despite not actually working there full time, I ended up spending most of my time there as it obviously became my gym. Also, as we had no money to pay coaches until we got more members, Daz would coach 90 per cent of the classes, so the other investors and I would help out when we could to give him a break, until we could afford to take on more coaches.

In March 2012, I did the first Open workout while attending a gymnastics seminar in Texas. The only real positive to come from the seminar was that I managed to improve my handstand walk but the other stuff they did like bounding (a type of box jump where you leap down and immediately back up again) was just too painful for me. I tried but no amount of bravery was going to get me through that one.

Bearing in mind I hadn't been able to run since November, the writing had already been on the wall for some time. I managed to complete the workout in Texas – 7 minutes of burpees – and my score was good enough to place me in the top three. But I was in so much pain throughout.

Word about my injury got back to my coach, Karl Steadman, the owner and coach at another CrossFit Gym in Manchester where I sometimes went to train. He was also a Level One CrossFit Instructor so when I made the decision to have some proper programming done after the 2010 Games I contacted him and he offered to be my coach.

To the untrained eye it might not have been obvious that I had a problem, but to Karl and James Jowsey, my movement coach, it was quite obviously an existing problem getting worse. So when I returned to the UK they asked me to go and see them. I remember getting a text from Karl when I landed saying, 'Can we see you for a coffee?' and I replied, 'Yes, of course.' There was nothing unusual in his request so I thought nothing of it. In fact, I assumed that he and James would want to talk to me about the next workout and find out how the gymnastics seminar had gone. What raised my suspicions slightly was that when I arrived at the gym the only people there were Karl and James. I knew then exactly what they were going to say. It was like being found out, in a way. I'd been doing something stupid for a long time and after getting away with it for far too long I was finally being called out. It had to happen though, for my own good.

When I finally plucked up the courage to enter the gym, there was no 'hello' or 'how are you'. It was straight down to business.

'I'm sorry, Sam, but we're pulling you from the Games,' Karl said immediately.

As the words came out of Karl's mouth, I could feel my stomach start to lurch downwards. It was a dreadful sensation and one that I'll never forget. In a few weeks I was due to turn thirty and I'd persuaded myself, over a very long period of time, that if I was ever going to win the CrossFit Games it had to be this year! After all, a 31-year-old could never win the CrossFit Games, right? Despite being one of the new girls, I was already one of the oldest individual competitors on the circuit and, as much as we try to tell ourselves that age is just a number, there comes a time in every situation when that's simply no longer the case. Fortunately for me, that wasn't yet true but at the time I was adamant it was and I felt broken. That's why I kept on training, though. It felt like it was now or never.

The funny thing is that when I did train the pain used to go away. Well, almost. Whether that was psychosomatic or not I couldn't tell you but, as long as I warmed up correctly and put a knee sleeve on, I'd be fine. I couldn't run, of course, but I was training and that, without wanting to sound too dramatic, was my lifeblood. It still is, as a matter of fact.

This obviously sounds ridiculous but, even after all the above, I still had some way to go in accepting that I wouldn't be able to compete at the 2012 CrossFit Games and in some of my weaker moments I'd sit there and try to think up ways to circumnavigate my problem. It was obviously futile but my determination (or perhaps that should be desperation?) and will to succeed still managed to get the better of common sense occasionally. Bearing in mind I'm not a stupid person, it was like being possessed.

What makes this even more ridiculous is that from a pain point of view, outside the gym that is, it was now completely off the scale and my drives to and from work during this period are times I'd rather forget. As with CrossFit, I hadn't said a word to anybody at work about this problem and as a consequence I'd been putting myself through an unimaginable amount of pain. The pain was at its worst while I was in a sitting position and, because I lived in Manchester but still worked in Leeds, every trip to and from work would be purgatory. It was always worse after a shift as my knee had already been put through the mill, whereas beforehand I'd been lying in bed. When getting in the car after a shift I'd put the radio on full blast and literally scream my head off the whole way back. Sometimes, if the traffic was bad, I could be there for a couple of hours. It was just horrific and if I could erase that period from my mind I would do so quite happily.

The penny finally dropped shortly after the second Open workout was released. I remember as clear as day what it was: thirty reps each of snatches using increasing weights of 45lb/20kg, 75lb/34kg, 100lb/45kg and 120/54kg. When I saw the workout released online I'd almost forgotten about what had happened. I remember going to see Karl and saying something like, 'I could muscle snatch the first few weights, no problem,' obviously hoping that he'd turn around and say okay.

'No, Sam,' Karl said. 'You are not doing any of the workouts. From now on I'd like you to concentrate on nothing but your rehabilitation, okay?'

After sitting me down and talking me through it – again – Karl finally managed to persuade me that, by pursuing this madness, not only would I dent my overall confidence by continuing to put in substandard performances, but I'd be in serious danger of ruining my chances of ever winning the CrossFit Games. If ever there was something that was going to make me see sense and put things into perspective, that was it, and with a heavy heart I finally accepted the reality of the situation and I officially withdrew from the 2012 Open.

When the news got out that I was withdrawing, I received several requests for interviews and fortunately the majority of these were over the phone. Even then it was difficult holding things together, and while the person on the other end was busy asking the questions I was doing lots of breathing exercises and trying not to cry. The only interview I agreed to do that was to be filmed was for the official CrossFit website and, as soon as I said yes, I knew it was a mistake. Sure enough, when the camera started rolling and the interviewer started asking questions, my emotions began to bubble over. Managing to keep it together for the duration of that interview (it only lasted two minutes!) is definitely one of my proudest achievements. My eyes are a bit watery and my bottom lip quivers like jelly but you don't see any tears.

My biggest flaw when I started CrossFit was definitely my technique. As well as stamina, I had raw strength in abundance from training with the boys at work, and right from the start I could do things like strict pull-ups and heavy deadlifts no problem whatsoever. My movement patterns and my mobility, however, were absolutely shocking, which again reminds me of my spell doing ballet.

As an example – and there are many – during the final event of the 2011 CrossFit Games we were doing something called a sumo deadlift high pull. This movement is similar to a deadlift but you have to widen your stance and bring the grip inside your knees to facilitate a longer pulling motion. In this instance we were using a 72lb/33kg kettlebell and my technique, or rather lack of it, was mentioned by the commentators who said, and I quote: 'Some athletes such as Samantha Briggs use only their upper bodies to muscle the weight up, whereas more efficient athletes such as Julie Foucher and Annie Thorisdottir are snapping the hips and driving through the legs so the arms are just an afterthought.' The commentator had got it absolutely right, although they did have to follow it up by saying that somehow I'd managed to make it work as I was the overall leader! Despite that, I obviously didn't win the Games or make the podium that year, and having now done both I know for a fact that a lack of technique was the missing link. And getting my knee sorted, of course.

To be fair, nothing I'd really done prior to CrossFit had required a great deal of technique. Even with football, I was definitely what you'd call an old-fashioned kind of player – I was aggressive, fast to the ball and I would win tackles but I wasn't skilled at all.

It wasn't until after pulling out of the Open that we – as in me and my movement mechanics coach, James Jowsey – decided to take some action. My regular coach, Karl, had introduced me to James about a year before and so with time on my hands we were able to address the issue of technique. 'Let's strip everything back and start again,' James suggested. 'It's the only way you're going to progress and if we don't do it now it'll never happen.' It sounded drastic but that's exactly what was required so we got to work. Because I was rehabilitating I was able to give this my full attention and that was absolutely pivotal. Had I been living and training as normal, it would have been a huge inconvenience and the finished article, as in me with only marginally better technique, wouldn't have been up to the job. Technique is something you should learn, or at least start to learn, right at the very start of your journey so, whatever you do, don't leave it as late as I did.

My relationship with James has come full circle really. After becoming my movement mechanics coach (the hardest job in CrossFit at the time), he then became my regular coach and, after I gave him a few years off for good behaviour, we got together again about three years ago. As an athlete, James knows me better than anybody and he's worth his weight in gold.

Eventually I had a scan on my knee and was told that I'd fractured my patella. The bone scan showed that the fracture had started to heal but there was a fragment left over that could potentially cause me problems. After talking it through with a surgeon, I was told that there was no guarantee that the scar tissue caused by an operation would be any less painful than leaving the fragment in. So, after further deliberation, we decided to leave the fragment where it was and start work on my rehabilitation.

The most difficult thing I had to endure during my rehabilitation wasn't anything physical like you'd expect. It was not being able to compete at the 2012 CrossFit Games. That caused me a very different, but nevertheless a very upsetting kind of pain, and while the Games were taking place I had to do everything in my power to try to distract myself. Ironically, literally the day before the Games started I was given the all-clear to start squatting again. Talk about a bittersweet experience. I didn't know whether to laugh or cry.

Because CrossFit is so varied, there were still many elements I could do that allowed me to still train to some degree throughout this period of rehabilitation. It was also the perfect opportunity to start working with Sean Lind and improve my gymnastics skills, as I'd never done that as a kid. By the late summer I had the all-clear to start full training again. Honestly, it was like getting my life back. I couldn't stop smiling.

Then, in September, I was invited to take part in the inaugural CrossFit Invitational. This was basically a head-to-head between the USA and Europe and had come about when CrossFit co-founder Greg Glassman and his team had asked themselves what would happen if you pitched the fittest on earth against each other in two teams of six. As well as being held at the XL Arena in London, it was also being televised throughout Europe on Eurosport. The idea was to showcase CrossFit by pitching its best athletes against each other, so the fact that they still invited me even though I had not competed at the Games that year was an amazing gesture and it couldn't have come at a better time.

As a concept this opened all kinds of doors for me. Athletes who had normally only been accountable to themselves and their coaches were now accountable to each other. Naturally, as a self-confessed team player, I found this an attractive proposition. Individual strength and endurance were still important, but so were things like teamwork, strategy and communication.

The first experience I'd had previously with team events in CrossFit was back in 2010 at a competition called Divided We Fall. Our gym used to enter a team each year and when I was asked if I'd like to take part I obviously said yes. There aren't many things I turn down, especially when CrossFit's involved.

We managed to get our team to the final of the competition and for the final event each team member had to complete the same workout. I can't remember who did what and when, but the very last movement was muscle-ups. The rings were set very high to make sure all the athletes could use them, and, because some of the girls in the competition were small, they made a rule that the person who goes before would be allowed to assist the next person. There were four of us on the team and it was decided that Daz, who co-owns the gym with me in Manchester, should go after me in this event as muscles-ups are one of my best disciplines, whereas he struggles with them, so we felt this would give him more time. As well as being about 6 foot 3 inches tall, Daz must weigh at least 100kg (that's 15.5 stone), so he's a big lad.

Unfortunately, Daz ran into trouble early on and, after giving him some time to sort himself out, it became clear I needed to intervene. With the team in a good position and the clock ticking away, something had to happen, so without a care for my own personal safety I stepped up. It wasn't going to be pretty, but it was our only option.

Try picturing this: a 5-foot 6-inch woman who's fit to drop attempting to push a giant into the air while he grapples with two rings and tries to get a false grip. I must have spent five minutes with my head in between his butt cheeks but it was all for nothing. In fact, he probably only managed one muscle-up. From a spectator's viewpoint it must have been hilarious but from where I was standing it was anything butt – pardon the pun. I certainly won't forget that in a hurry.

At the same competition a year later Daz smashed all his muscle-ups, no problem, but then he faced rope climbs in the final. He tried, bless him, but after the second attempt I took him to one side for a quick word. Seconds later, Daz was shimmying up the rope like a monkey and we managed to hold on to third. To this day, only he knows what I said to make him climb and everybody who's heard the story assumes that I either barked at him or issued a threat: 'Get up there now or I'll confiscate your post-competition beers!'

Each team at the Invitational comprised three girls and three boys and, despite it being, at least on the face of it, a promotional venture, the athletes were treating it as anything but. One of the workouts was a team Amanda featuring snatches and muscle-ups, and a Swedish athlete called Numi Katrinarson and I managed to beat Rich Froning, who'd won the Games for the last two years running, and Julie Foucher. For somebody who'd been out of the loop for over six months that was a really special moment. As well as more time in the gym and more time competing, I needed confidence more than anything else. Beating two athletes of that stature, live on television, gave me a huge boost.

Despite our best efforts, the USA ended up winning that Invitational by a few points but I think everyone was in agreement that it had been a great occasion. From a personal point of view, not only had I won an event at the competition, but, more importantly, I'd come through it injury-free.

About two or three months after the Invitational, I decided to take a six-month sabbatical from the fire service and concentrate fully on trying to win the CrossFit Games. Working nights just really wasn't conducive to this. The idea first came to me way back in March after pulling out of the Open. As a way to keep myself motivated I promised that if I ever managed to get through my rehabilitation I'd take some time off and just go for it. I knew it was something I would have to save up for to make sure I was financially able to keep myself afloat without a wage, so I had to be sure I was all in before I approached my bosses.

I remember actually making the decision to do it. The sensation I felt was the exact opposite to what I'd experienced when Karl had pulled me out of the Open. Then, my stomach had lurched southwards. This time it was going north with the rest of me.

In hindsight, there was actually no guarantee that the fire service would grant me a sabbatical, but I applied with plenty of notice and put together a well-thought-out case to support why I should be granted it. Fortunately, it was granted, and so, with the blessing of my colleagues and those closest to me, I began a journey that would ultimately becoming the making of me.

CHAPTER 15:

IT'S ALL IN THE PREPARATION

The first thing I had to do after being granted a sabbatical, which would start in March 2013, was to find some sponsors. As I've already said, the commercial side of proceedings is not my forte but with money being an essential ingredient to me being able to follow my dreams I had to change that pretty quickly. Luckily, I'd been saving, which helped, and already had a few sponsors on board at the time, but it was nowhere near enough. Fortunately, with a lot of help from friends and family, I finally managed to get enough support to see me through the six months. What a relief! With that now sorted, I was able to concentrate fully on preparing to become a professional athlete. It was a pretty terrifying prospect really, but in a good way. While I wouldn't say I was obsessed with my age, the old '*Can somebody over thirty ever win the CrossFit Games?*' question was still playing on my mind and one way or another I just had to answer it.

The night before the start of the 2013 Open, which began in March, I worked my last night shift as a firefighter. This meant that when I kicked off the 2013 CrossFit season I'd do so, for the very first time, as a full-time athlete. It's hard to find the words to express just how important this event was going to be. After all, this was to be my comeback, and most importantly, it was going to be my first individual test in CrossFit for over a year. Although nervous, I was up for the challenge.

This was the first year that CrossFit HQ decided to announce the workouts for the Open by pitching two athletes from each category against each other and then beaming it live to the world. These live demonstrations have now become a staple part of the proceedings and they're actually more like events really. The two individual girls chosen to compete for the final week of the Open were me and Camille Leblanc-Bazinet and the workout in question, although we didn't find that out until shortly before we started, was as many reps as possible in 4 minutes of fifteen 65lb/30kg thrusters and fifteen chest-to-bar pull-ups. If ninety reps (three rounds) were completed in under 4 minutes, the time extended to 8 minutes; and if 180 reps (six rounds) were completed in under 8 minutes, the time extended to 12 minutes and so on.

When I got the call to go I was thrilled to bits; not only because it made me feel like they still remembered me at CrossFit HQ but also because it meant a free trip to California, and I love California!

Every workout I'd ever done for the Open previously had been in a gym with maybe two or three people present. So, when I got the location of the workout, I was more than a bit surprised. Basically, it was an arena holding about 2,000 people and right in the middle of the floor was a platform where the workout would take place. It was a privilege being invited to take part in such a historic event and I couldn't wait to get started.

As well as having an audience present, the athletes taking part were asked to choose a walkout song each. This obviously added to the competitive element of the proceedings and made it feel a bit like a boxing match. In the end I decided to go with a gentle little number called 'Smack My Bitch Up' by The Prodigy. Funny and fitting, all in one! At the dress rehearsal we all went through the motions and on hearing my chosen song Camille started dancing.

'Hey, I like it,' she said. 'What's it called, "Take My Picture"? Yeah, it's great!'

Camille then started singing along to the chorus of the song using the words 'take my picture' instead of 'smack my bitch up'.

'Camille,' I said. 'You've got the words wrong. It isn't called "Take My Picture"; it's called "Smack My Bitch Up".'

'Oh,' she said, slightly taken aback. There was no more singing after that!

It was obviously supposed to be a joke and, fortunately for me, everybody concerned took it as one. I think people were starting to get a taste of my sense of humour! That flipping mischievous streak of mine.

Despite my best efforts, Camille managed to get the better of me but I still managed to post a good score and ended up coming eighth in the world in that workout. At the party afterwards, Greg Glassman came up to me and said, 'You were never meant to win that workout, Sam.' I'd never met Greg before and I was taken by surprise. Because of Camille's size she was always going to have an advantage in the workout so I'm pretty sure he was commiserating with me. At least I hope he was. He might have been rubbing it in!

As it happens, in the first and second Open workouts that year I took third place, then I won the third and fourth ones, meaning that, even though I took eighth on that final workout, I'd actually won my first Open. Without a doubt, I knew I'd made the right decision going all in. I even started feeling grateful for the fact that 2012 had been a write-off as, ultimately, it had presented me with this opportunity to take a very big stride forward. Had the injury not flared up, I wouldn't necessarily have made that change, so as strange as it might sound I was grateful for my kneecap almost exploding, just as I was grateful to Karl and James for having the good sense to pull me out. I'm not sure I believe in fate but at the time it all felt like it was meant to be.

From week two of the Open I took the overall lead and fortunately I managed to hang onto that lead and finish first in the world. Psychologically, this was a huge win as it validated everything I'd done over the past year and declared my intentions. Not just to those closest to me, but to the CrossFit community in general. I obviously wasn't going to win everything going forward, but to start 2013 with a resounding win in a global competition was significant to say the least. Now, as well as enjoying the fruits of my labours, I had to try to use it as a springboard going forward.

As you might expect, I went into the 2013 European Regional with a spring in my step. It took place in Copenhagen and when I arrived it appeared I wasn't the only athlete coming back from a knee injury. Finland's Mikko Salo was also making his return after having had a knee operation and to complete the coincidence he was also a fellow firefighter. The only difference between our situations was that Mikko had already won the Games, whereas I had yet to make the podium, but the fact that we were both making a return after injury seemed to cause quite a bit of interest within the CrossFit community.

The first of the seventeen CrossFit Regionals was, hopefully, going to be a good one. Unfortunately, the reigning CrossFit champion, Annie Thorisdottir, had to drop out with a back injury and, as regrettable as that undoubtedly was, at least it left the door open for someone new to lift the crown. The question was, who?

Out of the seven workouts, which included 'Jackie', featuring a 1,000-metre row, fifty thrusters and thirty pull-ups, I managed to win four and come third in the remaining three. Without wanting to sound like a big-head, that was a convincing win for me and the only slight downside, as mentioned by the commentator, was that Annie wasn't competing. We were considered to be two of Europe's best CrossFit athletes at the time and, with me not competing the previous year and her not competing on this occasion, it meant we'd have to wait until at least 2014 before we met again. Like me, it was important for Annie to make a full recovery before coming back and the timing was just unfortunate.

Nothing pushes you harder, though, than strong competition. So, in May 2013, I decided to find myself a training partner. Preferably somebody who was established in CrossFit and who could help me make that final step onto the podium. If I could do the same for them, all the better, so with that in mind I started thinking about who I could approach. After a while I had the idea of finding somebody who'd made a lot of progress at the last Games and, after going through the results, I came up with Lindsey Valenzuela. Although I didn't know her well, I'd met Lindsey while training with Kristan Clever and so, without giving it any further thought, I dropped her a message on Facebook. To be honest, I had absolutely no idea what Lindsey's reaction was going to be so when she replied and said, 'Hell yeah, let's do it,' it was a big relief. And it was exciting.

Part of my thinking behind approaching Lindsey was that she majored in strength, whereas I majored in endurance. Providing we got on well, I figured that we should be able to push each other in different directions and bring each other on. It was certainly worth a try.

Before going out to train with Lindsey, who was based in California, I first went to train with Laura Phelps-Sweatt for a couple of weeks at CrossFit Conjugate in Cincinnati. CrossFit Conjugate is the home of a group of coaches who specialise in training powerlifters, and at the time Laura was arguably one of the strongest women on earth. I think she held something like eighteen world records across different weight categories then and was the first female to total eleven times her bodyweight, so in terms of status and ability, I'd gone straight to the top of the pile.

Working with such an experienced and successful powerlifter was another luxury that I wouldn't have been able to afford had I not been a full-time athlete. Actually feeling like a professional athlete is just as important and empowering as being able to act like one, if that makes sense. It's a two-way thing and they obviously complement each other. Something that helped me to achieve the latter was having no distractions. In fact, I can't emphasise enough what a relief it was to be able to concentrate all my efforts on training.

There were definitely certain aspects of the fire service I missed, but apart from the people and camaraderie, the majority of these were training-related so there was nothing I hadn't either swapped like-for-like or improved on, really. However, I definitely missed the money – I wasn't being paid by CrossFit and, although I had gained a few sponsorship deals, the money wasn't rolling in. To save money during my stay with Laura I relied on the CrossFit community; fortunately, a member of Laura's gym, Bethany, offered to put me up and we soon became close friends.

When it came to my month-long stay with Lindsey, the plan was for me to stay with her and her family, so in terms of things that could go wrong the risk was pretty high for both of us. What if we didn't get on? What if we didn't train well together? What if she thought I was a loser? Looking back, it was actually quite a bold proposition and, had I been a more considered individual, I probably wouldn't have done it.

Fortunately, from the moment I arrived at Lindsey's house in Los Angeles I knew that everything was going to be okay and sure enough it was. In fact, it was better than okay, a lot better. Although we are opposites in almost every way, Lindsey and I managed to make every single one of these opposites work for us and we got on like a house on fire. Whether it was done intentionally or not I couldn't tell you, but what enabled us to make use of our differences was the fact that each of us had the same ultimate ambition – to win the 2013 CrossFit Games.

Just as important to the success of this 'experiment' was Lindsey's trainer, Dusty Hyland. He's the co-owner of a very well-known gym called Dogtown CrossFit in Culver City and I'd heard a lot about him. The atmosphere at the gym was incredibly relaxed and that suited my personality. It also suited the situation, in that if you're not careful you can sometimes get carried away by the enormity of what you're training for. Dusty and Lindsey seemed to have taken that into account so, although we all worked incredibly hard, we did so with very big smiles on our faces. Looking back, they're some of the happiest times I've had training and it was perfect preparation for what was in store.

Even from a young age I had a need for speed and would often be found climbing on the neighbour's motorbike … obviously I had my learner plates on for safety!

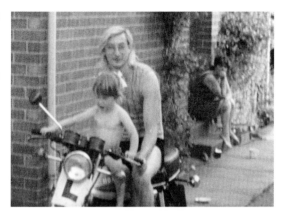

As you can see, me and my brother would regularly be matching … we loved our trips to the beach where we'd dig for hours.

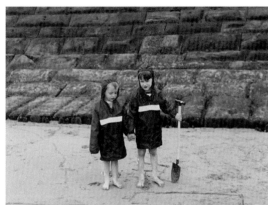

The only girl on the boys' football team.

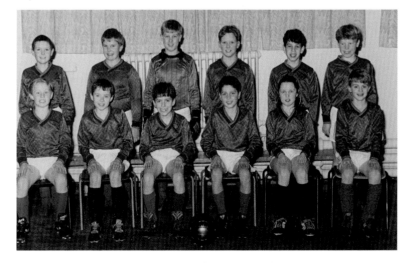

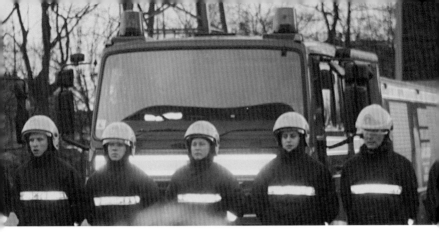

On parade with the rest of the 2004 recruits passing out after our three months' residential training … about to go out to the station and find out what it takes to be a real firefighter.

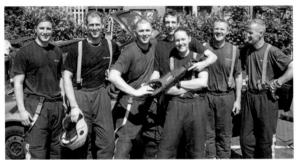

Me and the boys at Hunslet Fire Station striking a pose after some RTC training.

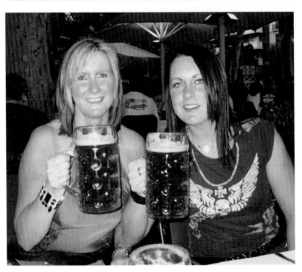

Me and my mum enjoying a small beer on one of our family holidays.

Trying my best to be a triathlete ... only to become stuck in my wetsuit!

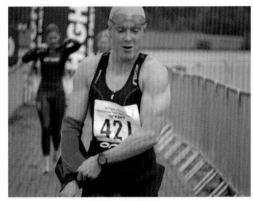

100kg-Daz carrying me in the partner carry relay before the roles reversed and I spent ten minutes picking him up to try help him get a muscle up!!

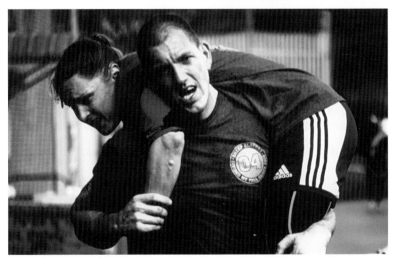

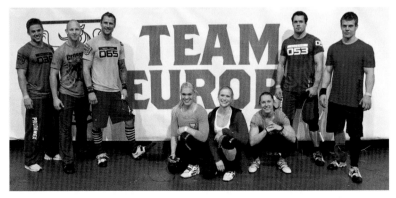

Team Europe getting ready for the first ever CrossFit Invitational.

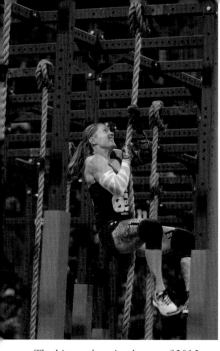

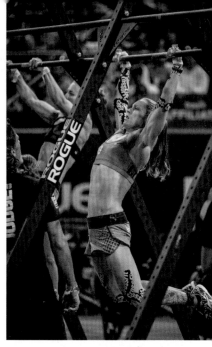

The biggest learning lesson of 2013 … never race a spider monkey.

2013 was a brutal year and thankfully my body was being held together nicely with lots of kinesio tape!

A dream come true! All the hard work and sacrifice had paid off.

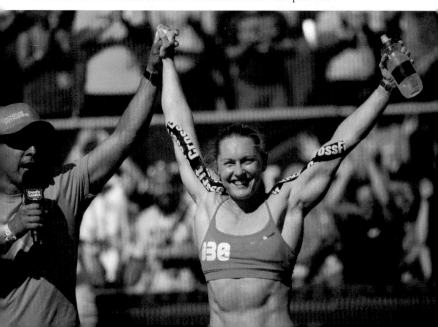

2015 Murph – the scorching California heat had lasting effects on many athletes!

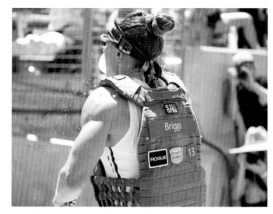

2016 Regionals and as happy as can be to be punching my ticket back to the Games.

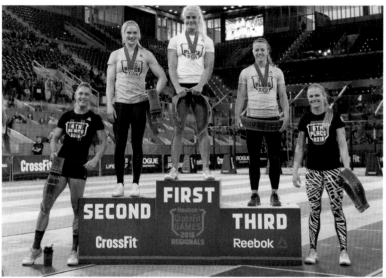

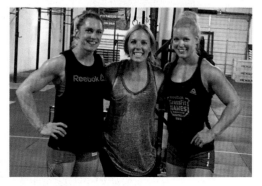

Pre-wedding workout with my friend Bethany and Nicole … even on your wedding day you've still got to get some fitness in.

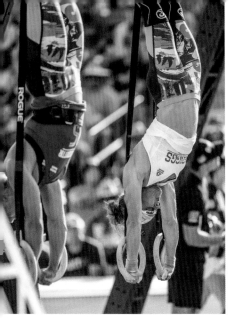

2016 Games – they threw some real challenges in for my shoulder … luckily adrenaline got me through the most complex of movements!

Getting ready to go head-to-head against Kristin Holte in Paris… we were still in good spirits despite it being 2am!

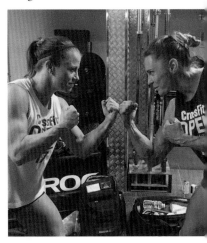

One of the things I'm thankful for from CrossFit are the opportunities to travel and see places I would probably have never ventured to … here we are hiking in Hawaii to raise money during the charity Ultimate Hawaiian Trail run.

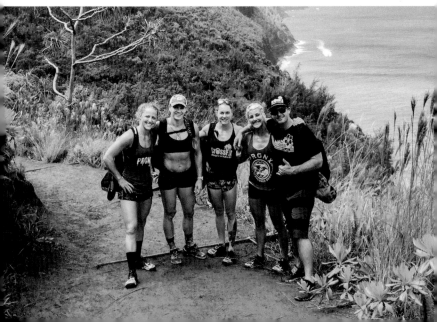

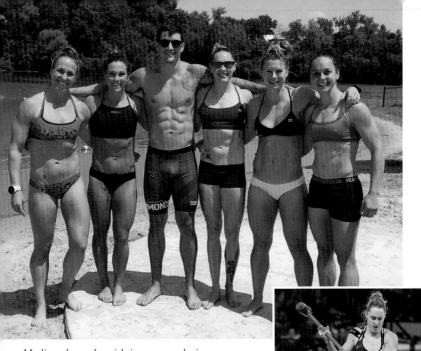

Madison brought with it a more relaxing setting for the Games preparations.

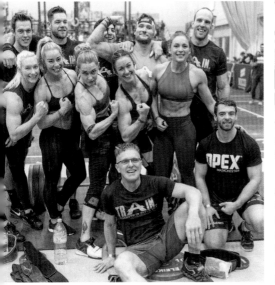

The Assault Banger workout allowed me to push through the limits and steal a win!

At the time, having to move back to the UK was devastating … but it did mean I got to spend more time at my gym TRAIN and compete regularly on a team with them.

Being back in the UK also meant I got to spend more time with my family and get my mum to train with me!

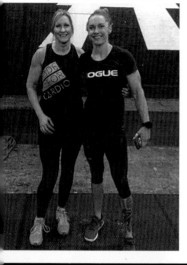

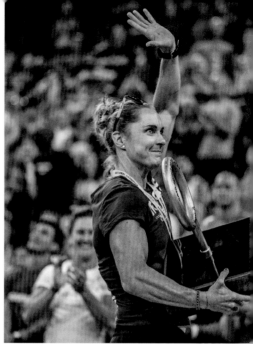

Being awarded the Spirit of the Games in 2019 is an achievement I doubt I'll ever be able to eclipse.

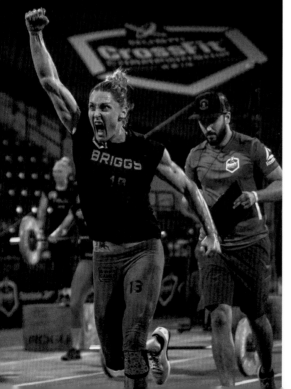

After a disappointing start to the 2020 season, I found my groove again and punched my ticket back to the Games in Dubai.

CHAPTER 16:
THE GREATEST DAY

By the time the Games came around I was in a really good place and that was obviously down to the previous few weeks. Having the freedom to think seriously about preparing for a competition was a luxury I was keen to hang onto and as I've got older that hasn't changed. In fact, it's something I take even more seriously.

One of the things I'd needed to think about beforehand was my support team. Because my coach from the UK was on the judging staff again, I didn't have anyone in my corner, so to speak, so a friend of mine volunteered to step in. As well as keeping me hydrated and giving me protein shakes, etc., he was also in charge of making sure I warmed up at the right time, so knowing that was all sorted was a big relief and helped me concentrate on the job at hand. Thanks, Dicko.

So now, with everything in place, all I had to do was wait to see what the CrossFit team had in store for us this year ...

Workout number one at the 2013 CrossFit Games, which took place on the Wednesday morning, was a pool event going for ten rounds for time of a 25-yard/23-metre swim, three bar muscle-ups and another 25-yard swim. I knew the moment I found out that this wasn't going to be my strongest event with the swim but ten rounds meant it would start to come into my domain, so I was confident of finishing well, and finish well I did. Fourth, in fact.

Workout number two was a half marathon row split into two. The first part, which was 2,000 metres for time, had 100 points riding on it so you had to go hard. Go in too hard, however, and the 21,097 metres left would obviously be a problem. I managed to finish joint first in Row 1 and won Row 2 so I must have judged it quite well. The main difference between my performance and the rest of the pack, although this definitely isn't advisable, was that after the row everyone else was having their quads, backsides or backs iced, whereas the only part of my body that needed any attention were my biceps. I think I rowed the entire thing with my arms!

People who know me will testify to the fact that, when I'm doing a workout, I always manage to stay focused. As a skill it's obviously invaluable in CrossFit and on several occasions over the years it's probably been the difference between me winning and losing. What might surprise you then, is that the only time I let my focus fall on someone else was on day two of the 2013 CrossFit Games. I still shudder when I think about it and with very good reason.

The third and final workout of day two, which was the Friday, was called 'Legless' and featured a mixture of legless rope climbs and thrusters. When the workout was announced I remember being quite pleased as it was something I did a lot and was good at. I'd even trained them with a weighted vest. Whether it was overconfidence or just madness that made me do this I'm not sure, but another athlete, Talayna Fortunato, was also quite proficient on a rope. Instead of ignoring that fact and just concentrating on myself, I decided to race her. At the CrossFit Games?! Incidentally, Talayna's nickname is Spider Monkey and when we started she had the same idea and came out as hot as I did. I still to this day don't know what made me do it. Jealousy of her having a cool nickname, perhaps? Who knows?

Consequently, we both started far too quickly and, instead of finishing the workout with a good time each like we should have, we actually failed on the same rope. We literally got within centimetres of touching the beam but unfortunately that last bit of grip strength just wasn't there. This moment of madness ended up dropping me from the top of the rope as well as from first place to second by the end of day two and to say that I was disappointed in myself would be a massive understatement. I was furious! I was just four points behind the leader, but that wasn't the point. I'd let myself down. The pressure you feel during the CrossFit Games is obviously immense so the fact that I'd actually added to that pressure was just ridiculous.

When I got back to the hotel I was feeling no better and I didn't sleep at all well. What I was in danger of doing at this point was allowing it to spoil my entire competition, so after waking up on the Saturday I decided to forget about what had happened and just concentrate on regaining the lead. In fact, by the end of the day that was my goal.

Lindsey Valenzuela and I had hotel rooms next to each other and on the Saturday morning, having had a below-average night's sleep coupled with a series of long days of early-morning briefings and late-night finishes, I remember saying to her half-jokingly, half-serious: 'Lindsey, I'm tired now, I don't want to play any more. I want to go home!' I was fine once we got to the athletes' briefing but that first half an hour or so before the adrenalin kicked in was hard work.

The first event on the Saturday was 'Naughty Nancy', which was four rounds for time of 600-metre run, up and over berm (an uphill/downhill run on steps around the stadium) and twenty-five overhead squats with a 95lb/43kg weight. Going into the workout, Christy Phillips was first on the leader board and I was in second, so my sole aim in the workout was to beat Christy. I figured that she was going to have the edge on me in the overhead squats so I had to make it count with the run.

I came out fast but not too fast and after going into the overheads marginally in the lead I thought I was in with a real chance. Kaleena Ladeairous ended up winning the event but she was outside the top ten and with Christy finishing mid-table I was back into first. Yes!

The second event on the Saturday was a clean and jerk ladder – one clean and jerk every 90 seconds with progressively heavier barbells. Not known for my strength, I had to settle for twenty-second place in this event. Fortunately for me, the only athlete in the top five or six to make it to the final bar was Lindsey, so despite her grabbing 95 points I still went into the last workout of the day in the lead.

The workout in question was a '2007' chipper comprising of a 1000-metre row followed by five rounds of twenty-five pull-ups and seven push jerks. At the time I was doing a 1000-metre row in the gym at about 1:45 pace; in other words, it would take me 1 minute and 45 seconds to row 500 metres. However, during this event, having already rowed a half marathon on the first day, I could not get my pace to drop to below 1:50. In the end I had to settle for a 2-minute pace and fortunately that was enough to see me leave the rower first.

I think Christy Phillips and Alessandra Pichelli were in second and third positions at this point and once again my goal was to keep ahead of them. In my two previous appearances at the CrossFit Games I'd been somewhere down the leader board so had always been fighting to get higher. Yes, there was pressure, but it was nothing like this.

Holding onto a lead is arguably the most pressurised situation an athlete can find themselves in. Sure, it's more desirable than playing catch-up, but as the one with everything to lose it's nerve-wracking beyond belief. Don't get me wrong, I was over the moon to be in that position, and wouldn't have wanted to swap it with anyone!

When I arrived back at the hotel I went to my room and tried to collect my thoughts. As well as being in first position I was now just one day and three workouts away from being crowned 2013 CrossFit Champion and the fittest on earth. It was, as the popular cliché goes, mine to lose. Once again, sleep didn't come easily but I do remember having a dream that night so I must have got some. The dream featured me, Lindsey and Val Voboril and all I could really remember was that the three of us were on the podium. This wasn't just a dream, it was a flipping wish list.

When I woke up I felt tired but excited. I remember switching on my phone before leaving for the briefing and there must have been at least twenty messages from people all wishing me well. I hadn't been expecting them so it was a really nice surprise. A close friend of mine had asked me what my game plan was in one of the messages and I'll always remember how I answered it. 'Stay calm', I wrote, 'and don't mess up. That's my game plan.' In truth, it was actually more of a mantra really and throughout the morning I kept on whispering it to myself. Stay calm and don't mess up. Stay calm and don't mess up. My other strategy for coping, although this was slightly more tongue in cheek, was denying that it was happening at all. Nope, this isn't happening to me, I'd say. I am not leading the CrossFit Games. It's all a dream!

Had I known what the first workout of the day was going to be prior to leaving the hotel, I'd have felt a lot more trepidatious than I did and when the details were finally imparted to us I might just have whispered a rude word. 'Workout one will be a sprint chipper,' they said. 'For the individual women it will be twenty-one med-ball GHD sit-ups, fifteen snatches and nine wall burpees for time.' (GHD sit-ups, incidentally, are done on a glute-hamstring developer machine, which means you have to bend right back on the downward motion, raising a heavy medicine ball above your head.) Chippers are great for me, sprints not so much, so it was going to be interesting. My ideal time for a workout is ten minutes plus. In fact, the closest you can get to thirty minutes, the better. This one was going to be sub three minutes so, if ever there was a time to start proving people wrong, including myself, about me and sprint events, this was it. What changed things mentally for me was that this was going to be the last workout before the final and because we didn't know what that final event was going to be I had to give this first workout everything I had.

After arriving at the stadium, one of the first things I saw on one of the big screens was the current leader board. Nine out of the twelve athletes had American flags to the left of their names and the athletes lying in tenth and twelfth had Australian and New Zealand flags respectively. There was only one Union Jack and that, fortunately, was still at the very top of the leader board. I remember thinking, *Let's just hope it stays there!* Incidentally, I was on 672 points going into the final day. Alessandra was on 637 and Valerie Voboril and Christy Phillips were on 602. It wasn't a done deal by any means, but it was still a good lead.

Kristan Clever won the first heat with a time of 3:02.3 and the winner of heat two, Camille Leblanc-Bazinet, smashed that time by over 20 seconds by posting 2:41.4. For heat three I was in lane eight in between Valerie Voboril and Alessandra Pichelli and the two favourites were Valerie and Christy Phillips, who were joint third. First to the second movement was Alessandra, who quickly managed to build up a 2-rep lead over Michele Letendre and Jenn Jones. A lot of athletes started to tire about this point and the first three athletes to the burpee wall were Jenn Jones, Lindsey Valenzuela and – shock horror – Samantha Briggs! What I was doing that far up the field I have absolutely no idea but I was certainly pleased to be there. I remember hearing the commentator counting Jenn's reps and because she was in the lead I listened carefully and did my best to keep up. I lost track of the commentator somewhere along the way so just went for it and when I finished my final burpee and started sprinting for the line the only other athlete with me was Jenn. Nobody was more surprised by this turn of events than I was and, when I ended up crossing the line with a time of 2:35.03, just three-tenths of a second ahead of Jenn, I was absolutely elated.

After watching it back, I could see I started getting the better of her on the very last climb and fortunately I was able to get ahead and maintain my lead. Just! I remember being interviewed afterwards in front of the crowd and, after being asked by Amanda Krenz how I was feeling and what I had to do to win the final two workouts, I all but repeated my mantra from the morning. Stay calm and don't make any mistakes! I also said that I would be happy with any position on the podium, but that was a great big fib. I had come here to win the Games and, going into the final in the lead, anything other than the top step was going to be a disappointment for me.

To put it into perspective, all I needed from the last two events was about 135 points, which was the equivalent of finishing in the top seven or eight in each. I may not have been the favourite for the last two events but neither was I an outsider. So, providing I held my nerve and 'didn't make any mistakes', I was sure I'd be okay. The biggest danger at this point was either getting injured or not finishing one of the events. Had the latter happened at the first event, then I'd have had to finish in front of Alessandra in the final event, or something like that. There were so many possibilities going into the final and it was one of those situations where I had to listen to what was truly important to me – winning – and let everything else just disappear.

Alessandra was the new girl on the block. In 2012, her debut year, she'd finished 312th in the Open, third in the team event at the Regionals and then third at the Games. In 2013, she'd finished eighth at the Open and first at the Northern California Regional, so she was obviously a contender to win the Games and I think everyone had an eye on her. Because of how her career had gone so far, in the way that she'd managed to carry the momentum of having a decent debut year at the Games into year two, the two of us had been compared by a couple of commentators.

The two final workouts of the 2013 CrossFit Games were called 'Cinco 1' and 'Cinco 2'. Cinco 1 consisted of three rounds of five deadlifts (265lb/120kg) and five weighted one-legged squats on the left leg and then on the right leg, followed by an 80-feet/24-metre handstand walk. The only part that concerned me were the one-legged weighted squats, for the simple reason that they're one of the hardest movements on the knee and my knee obviously wasn't my strongest body part. If a disaster was going to happen, this was probably where it would take place. I remember trying a couple in the transition area and thinking, *That'll do, Samantha … save them for the workout!*

The time limit for the workout was just 7 minutes and, after either completing the workout or running out of time, you then had a 1-minute rest before Cinco 2. Sound easy? Well, Cinco 2 was even worse. That was three rounds of five muscle-ups and five deficit handstand push-ups (where you do your handstand push-ups on portable raised parallel bars on the floor – parallettes – meaning you have to lower yourself below the bars on the downward motion) followed by a 90-foot/27-metre overhead walking lunge carrying a 100lb/45kg axle bar. Again, we had 7 minutes to complete this workout.

Before being introduced to the crowd, the athletes had to gather in the tunnel out of sight. I remember standing there trying not to look nervous and then realised that the other nine athletes were doing exactly the same! We all failed miserably, by the way. The biggest cheers between athletes ten and two went to Lindsey and Valerie who are both Californians. That made me feel really good. Then it was my turn.

'Lane 5, in first place,' said the commentator, 'from Manchester, England ... Sam Briggs!'

Despite there being about twenty people from the UK in the crowd and three or four Union Jacks, I was expecting a warm reception rather than a raucous one. After all, the rest of the 25,000 spectators were probably American, so why go crazy for an English girl? Talk about a surprise. As I ran out and waved to the crowd they just erupted. What a boost! It's something I'll never, ever forget.

After reaching my lane, we had one minute to prepare for the workout. It felt more like five seconds! Lindsey was quickest out of the blocks and, when I watched the video, she makes the deadlift look easy. Then again, she did have a max deadlift of almost 400lb/180kg at the time so it would have felt a lot lighter to her than some of the others. Me included.

First onto the handstand walk was Christy Phillips, who ended up crossing the line in second position behind Talayna Fortunato. Next up were Valerie and Lindsey who finished third and fourth respectively. The two athletes vying for fifth were me and Alessandra, and I knew that if I beat Alessandra, barring a disaster, I'd have all but won the Games. Although I ended up beating Alessandra by a foot or two, I almost threw it away as, instead of getting up and running across the finish line having completed the handstand walk, I forgot about the last bit and started celebrating. Fortunately, I remembered just in time but it could have cost me.

The next thing I remember is staring up at the muscle-up rings and hearing the words 'ten seconds' coming through the speakers. It's hard to describe how tired I felt at this point. It was as if everything had been magnified by ten: the heat, the exhaustion, the pressure. One final push was required but I had nothing left in the tank. Only adrenalin could get me through now.

The part of the workout that worried me most were the deficit handstand push-ups. They weren't that common in CrossFit at the time and took a lot of strength, which at that point in the competition everyone was struggling with. Sure enough, they were my undoing. Fortunately, I was able to keep up with my muscle-ups to get onto the lunges and I ended up tying with two other athletes in that heat, which put me in fourth place overall.

When the airhorn went to signify the end of the 7 minutes, the first thing I did was run over to Lindsey. I've made so many friends in CrossFit but Lindsey and I had shared so much together and the only thing that I was bothered about after the airhorn – apart from whether I'd won the CrossFit Games, of course – was if Lindsey had made it onto the podium. That was the only thing on my mind. We'd pushed and helped each other to such a degree that we were basically a team of two individuals.

Funnily enough, the biggest compliment I've ever been paid by a fellow athlete is when Lindsey was asked by an interviewer what it had been like training with me. This was either just before or just after the Games and she replied that she'd never known anybody care for other athletes as much as I did. I almost cried when I saw it. If CrossFit was all about the individual, it wouldn't work for me. Yes, I want to win. I want to win desperately. But I promise you, I get just as much satisfaction from seeing other people succeed and for me the two go together hand in hand. I'm only really doing well when those around me are doing well.

After speaking to Lindsey, I walked to the centre of the stadium floor and signed my time sheet. I'd love to see that signature again as I bet it's no more than an illegible squiggle! It's always the same after a competition. You're invariably shaking because you're exhausted but with what I'd just achieved I'm surprised I could lift the pen. The next thing I remember is looking in the crowd to find Mum. I should have known exactly where she was sitting really but at the time I was a little bit disorientated. In the end all I had to do was find the Union Jacks! After giving her a big wave, I spent a few moments just taking in the atmosphere. That's a moment I'll never forget for as long as I live. The sun was shining, and as well as being surrounded by 25,000 smiling people I was about to be crowned the fittest woman on earth. If somebody had suggested this to me when I'd arrived at my first CrossFit class four years ago, I'd have laughed them out of the building. How in heaven's name had this happened?

Just as I was taking a sip of water and trying to take it all in, Dave Castro, the director of the CrossFit Games who was standing about ten feet away from me, confirmed the result.

'Ladies and gentlemen,' he said, before walking over, taking my hand and holding it aloft. 'I give you your 2013 Reebok CrossFit Games champion ... Samantha Briggs!'

He used my full name!

The icing on the CrossFit cake was that Lindsey and Valerie had finished second and third respectively, so not only had my dream come true of winning the CrossFit Games, but my literal dream from the night before had also come true as my two friends would be joining me on the podium. For the presentation ceremony I had to go back into the tunnel and wait for my name to be called out. This time, though, instead of running out to lane five wearing a vest and shorts, I was draped in a Union Jack. Oh yes, I also had a very, very big smile on my face.

After soaking up the applause for a second and waving for all I was worth to my friends and family, I took my place on the podium next to my friends, Lindsey and Valerie. As I stood there, a million things started running through my head. The injury, the recovery, the hard work. Every day of my life since finally pulling out of the Open had been lived with one thing in mind, winning the CrossFit Games and becoming the fittest woman on earth. One thing's for sure, it was going to take time to sink in.

CHAPTER 17:

ME, ON *BBC BREAKFAST*?

The period after the CrossFit Games ended was strange. It was and still is a bit of a blur, as when you spend so long working towards something and eventually succeed it's sometimes a bit of a shock. And it doesn't matter how much self-belief you have. Realising a dream and/or defying the odds are not everyday occurrences and, although it was obviously a very special time, it's all a bit ethereal in my memory now.

With my visa fast running out I came back to the UK straight after the Games. This was quite a welcome turn of events as I was keen to share what had happened with those friends and members of my family who hadn't been able to make it to the Games. And also catch up on their news, of course.

When I arrived back, the only thing on my mind, apart from having good gossip, was having fun. It wasn't necessarily a conscious decision. Life had been so intense for so long and, now that it was all over, I think my attitude had shifted automatically from *Concentrate on the job in hand no matter what, Sam*, to *Sod it, you deserve a rest!* I obviously carried on training but, instead of going into the gym all day, I went in, did a workout for an hour and then trotted off to enjoy the rest of the day.

This lasted for a week or so, after which thoughts of my future started making an appearance. It was time to sit down and make a decision. Either I go back to work to continue with my career or I knuckle down and try to retain my title. Financially, I was actually doing okay. The prize money from winning the Games meant I could have some serious savings to fall back on and new sponsorship deals in the pipeline would put me in a good position.

All things considered, the decision took about five seconds and, just a few days after returning from the USA, I asked the powers that be at the fire service for an extension on my sabbatical. As always, they were incredibly supportive and said yes almost immediately. Despite winning the Games, I still didn't know if I could make a living out of CrossFit full time, so if I were a gambler I'd still have put money on me ending up doing both long term. Funnily enough, since getting back from America, several offers had been made that ultimately would go some way to helping me commit to CrossFit, but for now I just had to try to balance both worlds.

I was also asked to do some mainstream media interviews, which was interesting. Usually it was somebody from a CrossFit website or a fitness magazine who wanted to talk to me but now I'd won the Games I was being approached by the likes of *BBC Breakfast*. Well I never! My social media profile also went off the scale after the Games (it was mainly Facebook in those days) and I don't think I've ever had as many likes in my life. I've never been what you'd call an expert at social media as I prefer to do my talking either in the gym or face to face. Despite that, it obviously enables people to communicate on a massive scale and my usual aim when posting things is either to inspire people or make them smile. Hopefully I get it right sometimes.

The best thing to come from winning the CrossFit Games in an immediate sense – apart from happily slacking at the gym for a few days and appearing on breakfast telly – was being invited to take part in the 2013 CrossFit Invitational in Berlin in October. I'd already had experience of this event in the inaugural Invitational the previous year, and I was really excited about being able to take part in it again.

For 2013, the organisers had decided to open up the field, so instead of it being USA versus Europe it was going to be USA versus the Rest of the World. Or Team World, as we were known. Team USA consisted of Rich Froning, Jason Khalipa, Ben Smith, Lindsey Valenzuela, Valerie Voboril and Talayna Fortunato. Not bad, I suppose. On our side we had – girls first – Camille Leblanc-Bazinet representing Canada, Kara Saunders representing Australia and me representing Europe, and on the boys' side we had Frederik Aegidius (Europe), Chad Mackay (Australia) and Albert-Dominic Larouche (Canada). No disrespect to the boys on our team, but in those days the American male athletes dominated the sport, so, despite the female contingent being more than a match, the American team, on paper at least, definitely had the advantage.

Bearing in mind what I said earlier about Lindsey and Val, you might think it slightly strange me having to compete against them so soon after the Games but it was anything but. Despite our friendship and camaraderie, we'd only ever competed against each other so the fact that Lindsey and Val were on a different team to me didn't matter at the time. What also transcends everything is that when push came to shove we were all there for each other, regardless of what country or continent we came from. Trying to explain that to somebody who doesn't know CrossFit isn't easy as it's obviously paradoxical, but to those who do it's second nature.

I arrived in Berlin about a week before the competition and the buzz in the city was just incredible. In Los Angeles you obviously get something similar but here everything was in closer proximity, including the spectators. The competing athletes trained in a local CrossFit gym and towards the end of the week it was full to bursting; not just with the athletes who were competing, but with ordinary CrossFitters who had travelled from all over the world to watch the event. The Invitational took place at an old airport called Tempelhof and, as well as being a complete sell-out, it was also being televised live on Eurosport. In terms of popularity it was the closest thing Europe had to the CrossFit Games, I suppose, and taking it out of America, as they had also done last year, was a masterstroke. What captured the public's imagination most, however, was the team element.

Team World's biggest worry at this competition was that Team USA were stronger overall. The only member of their team who hadn't been on the podium at this year's Games was Talayna, and even she'd finished fifth. This meant that, on paper, Team USA had in their ranks five out of the six current fittest people on earth. We were definitely no slouches, but five out of six? It was a seriously daunting prospect.

In order to try to counter Team USA's potential advantage, we had to play a strategic game. This meant us trying to guess who they would put up for certain workouts and then attempting to use that to our advantage. For instance, because Lindsey was by far the best lifter, we were adamant that Team USA would put her up for the most points on the lift-off, and they did. The athlete she would be competing against in that was me and you already know she's a better lifter than I am. So why put me up? Well, with Lindsey out of the way, Kara and Camille were going to have a better chance of beating the other two girls, and fortunately this paid off. It was basically just a sacrifice. One loss for two wins.

These kinds of showcase events are fantastic to be involved in and the atmosphere in the converted hangar was amazing. There must have been about 5,000 spectators present and, because this was basically their CrossFit Games, they never stopped cheering from the moment we took to the arena floor.

Team World managed to win the first workout – 1000-metre row, fifty thrusters with an empty bar and thirty pull-ups – by eleven points to ten, and with Team USA being the odds-on favourites this immediately raised a few eyebrows. Then, after we girls won the female half of the second event – fifteen dumbbell burpee box jumps, thirty partner-deadlifts (when two athletes lift the same bar in tandem), thirty overhead squats and fifteen muscle-ups per athlete – we were in danger of causing an upset.

Luckily for us, the girls from Team USA just couldn't keep up with us on this workout. Kara and Camille were more proficient in the overhead squats but I managed to redeem myself on the deadlifts.

Unfortunately (or fortunately if you were either an American or a neutral spectator), Team USA won the next two workouts convincingly, which left everything to play for. We might not have been favourites to win the competition but as a team we were confident, not just in our own abilities, but in each other's.

Team USA went into the final event, which comprised of a 30-metre handstand walk, sixty team worm-thrusters (in which the team lines up single file to squat while lifting a huge wooden log, strung together with rope, above the head in unison) and a

30-metre overhead walking lunge, with a slender two-point lead. So, despite our confidence, order had been restored to the watching world and the USA were favourites once again.

A fitness magazine I read after the event summed up our performance in the handstand walk perfectly. They wrote: 'One could see that Sam Briggs had worked on her handstand walk, but Kara Saunders and Camille smashed it!' I couldn't have put it better myself. I think we regained the lead during the worm-thrusters. To the untrained eye this movement looks like a slightly bizarre party game for adults but as well as being incredibly punishing it's all about communication, synchronisation and teamwork. As far as I can remember we only had to take a break twice during this movement and by the time we moved onto the lunges we had a lead over Team USA of about twenty seconds.

Kara Saunders started off the lunges and we all followed. I remember watching Team USA as they carried the worm to the back of the arena after finishing their reps. They were absolutely done in, as were we. I watched a video of this bit a while ago and Kara's legs are literally shaking like jelly as she gets towards the finish and the look on her face made me think just one word – *help!*

Your team hadn't finished until every member had crossed the 30-metre line so, despite Kara having done her bit, there was still a way to go. By the time Camille crossed the line, Rich Froning, who was leading Team USA's charge, had caught me up, which meant, in terms of athletes finished, we had a lead of two. But for how long? With just two athletes to go – one on either side – it was between Chad Mackay and Valerie Voboril. Both were on the verge of collapse but, despite dropping the bar on the line, while Valerie was making up ground, Chad managed to complete his final lunge. In doing so he gave Team World an unexpected but nevertheless very welcome win at the 2013 CrossFit Invitational. I should mention that it was Kara Saunders' birthday on the day we won, which meant she was allowed the first swig of champagne!

In order to bring myself back down to earth after the Berlin Invitational, I decided to sign up for a powerlifting competition in December. Laura Phelps-Sweatt was holding one at her gym in Cincinnati and the reason I entered was just to show my support. Although obviously connected to my CrossFit training, the competition itself was going to be different to anything I'd experienced previously and I hoped it would be a contrast to the CrossFit juggernaut that had been dominating my life.

A day of competitive powerlifting couldn't be more different to a day of CrossFit and as the day began I found the pace of the competition very difficult to adjust to. With CrossFit you might do three or four workouts in a day and they could last from, say, three to forty-five minutes apiece. The pace is usually quite frenetic both before, during and in between the workouts. I perhaps hadn't appreciated it but that was a big part of the attraction for me. I like to crack on with things!

With powerlifting you'll do three lifts in one day and you'll have three attempts at each lift. There's a break of about fifteen minutes in between each attempt and a two-hour break in between each lift. That was the bit that I couldn't get used to. It was torture! You see, as well as having the attention span and the boredom threshold of a hyperactive five-year-old child, my body tends to seize up if I don't do anything for more than about fifteen minutes. I just have to keep moving! As a consequence, instead of resting in between each lift I decided to go backstage and do intermediate lifts. Well, it seemed like a good idea at the time.

Most of the powerlifters were using smelling salts throughout the day and, although I was offered some, I declined. I couldn't see the point in sniffing something that seemed to make people recoil in disgust. By the time we got to the final lift, which was the deadlift, I was so tired I relented and asked for some smelling salts. Having done at least fifty more lifts than I needed to, it was no surprise I was knackered. I have to say that the smelling salts were a revelation and if it hadn't been for them I definitely wouldn't have been able to deadlift that last bar. Effectively the ammonia gives you a temporary adrenalin rush, which dulls the pain in your muscles. I was so tired by the deadlift that I took no intermediate lifts backstage; instead I just collapsed into a heap between my attempts, waiting for my name to be called again. For my bodyweight, my bench and my deadlift were pretty competitive, but my squat let me down, so I was more than happy to finish third in my class.

Despite the difference in pace, I did actually enjoy lifting and felt being on the platform would only help my CrossFit career. So I decided to enter the Northern Open Olympic Lifting Championships that year too. I ended up winning in my category, meaning I had qualified for the English Championships. The thing is, I'd qualified in the 63kg category and had I stayed there I'd have been competing against athletes like Zoe Smith. Even at the age of nineteen, which is what she was then, Zoe was already a Commonwealth Games medallist and held several British records. It was by far the most competitive category in the women's competition, so to give myself a chance of medalling I decided to slim down to the 58kg category. This turned out to be a bit of a masterstroke and, although I missed my first two snatches, I came through on the third and after getting all three clean and jerks I managed to get first place. I was the English champion! That was a pretty good end to what had been an extraordinary year. And after dropping weight I could have a huge celebratory meal!

CHAPTER 18:

PULLING THE LADDERS UP

Apart from the Invitational, one of the most interesting offers to land immediately after the Games was for an event called the Immortals CrossFit Challenge. It was at the time Australia's leading team CrossFit competition and was being held somewhere in the Gold Coast on 9 and 10 November. One hundred teams of six would be taking part and they'd be littered with Regional-level CrossFit athletes as well as six or seven from the CrossFit Games. It was also held to raise money for charity, so I was in!

One of the reasons I was so keen on going – apart from it being another team event, which I enjoyed, and getting a free trip to Australia of course – was because I'd be competing alongside a friend of mine called Nicola Smith. As well as being a former Great Britain rugby league player and Muay Thai boxing champion, Nicola was also an accomplished CrossFit athlete and she'd finished fourth at this year's European Regionals. Not only had we trained together a lot but we'd also got on really well. What made the proposition even more attractive was that the third and final girl on our team would be Talayna Fortunato who I'd just competed against at the Invitational. With three decent Regional-level men, Jonnie Larmore, Dean Linder-Leighton and Marcus Smith, completing our team, I was hopeful of continuing my post-Games winning streak and couldn't wait to get out there.

Held over two days and in memory of fallen soldiers, the Immortals CrossFit Challenge featured five workouts on day one and the reason I'm going to list them is that it gives you an idea of how things change and work at team events:

Workout 1

For time – one boy and one girl work at once through a 12-9-6 rep scheme of overhead squats (60kg for men and 40kg for girls) and burpee box jumps.

Workout 2

All six team members file through in Indian file featuring fifteen pull-ups, fifteen toes-to-bar, fifteen wall-balls, fifteen toes-to-bar, fifteen pull-ups and repeat as many times as you can for 10 minutes.

Workout 3

Girls and boys are split and, while two of the team row for calories, one pushes a 100kg sled for 15 metres. The team then rotates after 10 minutes.

Workout 4

Boys start on the Airdyne (a cycling machine) and go for 5 minutes maximum calories while the girls go for maximum med-ball slams with a 20kg ball. After 5 minutes they rotate and the boys use a 30kg ball.

Workout 5

Two boys flip a wombat (a huge metal bar with chunky weights at either end) twice and then the girls flip it once until it reaches the 20-metre line. Then it is flipped back to the other end with the girls flipping twice and the boys once.

My team, called Team Innerfight, won three out of the five events on the first day so it was a great start. On day two the teams were split into three categories – beginner, intermediate and elite – with the workouts being scaled accordingly. The idea behind this was to allow all levels of competitors to be involved right up to the final.

The workouts for day two were as follows:

Workout 1
In pairs: 12-9-6 deadlift, hang power clean, push jerk, 80kg for the boys and 50 kg for the girls.

Workout 2
50 bar muscle-ups between the team. Then, in mixed pairs: 40 burpee box jump overs, 30 push jerks followed by a maximum distance row. Time cap of 15 minutes.

For the final event, instead of a team workout it would be a relay-style workout; then to keep thing interesting they made it a winner-takes-all affair with all the previous scores being wiped.

So the following workouts were done back to back with one team member doing one element before the next person started their part:

15 calories on the Airdyne
'Fran': 21-15-9 thrusters, pull-ups
30 clusters at 70kg (this is a clean that goes into a thruster)

30 fat bar deadlifts at 100kg, 30 bar-facing burpees
150 wall-balls
One length of the arena flipping the wombat @ 240kg

Day two kicked off with the top ten teams going for the first workout and we managed to take this home with yet another first place. We needed to stay in the top five to make the final, and in the second workout of the day we finished as runners-up by less than 50 metres on the rowing machine. Runners-up or not, we were in the final.

After the Airdyne we were lying fifth but, with Talayna setting an all-time personal best of 2:06 on Fran, Dean Linder-Leighton went into his squat clean thrusters in third place. Once Dean was done it was over to Jonnie Larmore who went through the deadlifts and burpees like a flash before tagging me. The only time I paused was with fifteen reps to go, by which time I'd managed to build up a sizeable lead on the rest of the field. My legs were fine. It was just my arms that seemed to give out but I got there in the end. On tagging Marcus Smith I had a feeling that he was going to make mincemeat of the wombat and I was right. His attitude was anything but casual, however, and as he crossed over the finish line we were over two minutes ahead of the second-placed team.

In terms of profile, the win was obviously on a different scale to the Invitational but it had been no less enjoyable. I'd visited a new country, had made new friends and I'd been involved in a competition that had raised a lot of money for charity. What's not to like? Well, there was a downside to my trip, unfortunately, although it had nothing to do with the competition or its organisers.

After I confirmed my attendance, the original contact who had first told me about the event then asked if I'd be interested in delivering an instructional seminar while I was over there. As somebody who very much enjoys banging the CrossFit drum, I said I'd do it, as did the other athletes. We understood that we would do one seminar to help with costs and then the rest of the trip would be paid for in return for us doing some media work.

The guy drove us around for the beginning of the trip and everything seemed legit – at first. But then we discovered we were expected to go to more and more gyms, and when we got there it transpired the members were expecting a seminar that they had paid for upfront! When we discovered this we confronted the guy and found out that there was no media work and instead he had been taking money from people for seminars we knew nothing about.

In the end we tried to honour as many of the seminars as possible, though we cut all our ties with the guy and I'd be happy to never see him again! Unfortunately, this man had also booked some seminars at a few gyms in Sydney and, given we were based in Brisbane, there was no way we could honour them. Not without a magic carpet! This was the most disappointing aspect, as, although it wasn't our fault, there was bound to be guilt by association. All people would remember was that Samantha Briggs hadn't turned up to a seminar. That really didn't sit well with me. I didn't want to let the people down who had paid money and were expecting a service from me, plus I enjoyed instructing people and passing on CrossFit. It just meant that we had to cancel our sightseeing and spent most of the remaining days in the gym instead.

There was nobody we could really complain to about this as foolishly we hadn't signed a contract. All this was new to us and so far everyone associated with CrossFit had been super friendly, so it hadn't occurred to us to be wary. As we'd cut ties with him I was slightly worried that he'd not booked or would cancel my flight home from Australia and when it came to going home I was half expecting the airline to say, 'I'm sorry, madam, but your seat hasn't been paid for.' It wouldn't have surprised me. Fortunately, it was all okay and I got home safely.

Seminars in Sydney notwithstanding, 2013 had obviously been a pretty good year for me and I went into 2014 full of aspiration. Saying that, you're only ever as good as your last win so there were no laurels for me to rest on. Also, on 14 March 2014 I was going to be thirty-two years old. When I won the CrossFit Games I'd been something like eleven years older than the youngest finalist and my age had been commented on by so many people. It hadn't been an issue, exactly. More of a feature, if anything. *Here comes Sam Briggs. Isn't it amazing how she can perform like this in her thirties?!* The thing is, I didn't want to be judged by my age. Nothing's changed in that department. I want to be judged purely on my ability and, if I happen to be a bit older than some of my competitors, so what? Nobody likes being reminded that they're older than the people they work alongside, least of all an athlete.

In the spring of 2014, I was told that the fire service were making budget cuts. This meant that every firefighter on a sabbatical was going to be recalled and the truth was I didn't want to be recalled! Although I still wasn't sure if I could make a career out of CrossFit, I was having far too much fun and success to let the dream slip away, so with my hand now being forced I decided to make the break and hand in my notice. With the decision being all but made for me, the anxiety I'd been harbouring about it just slipped away and I was left with what I hoped would be a bright future.

Had CrossFit not come along, I'd have happily stayed in the fire service for the rest of my working life. Then again, had I not joined the fire service, the chances are I wouldn't have found CrossFit. In every respect, my ten years in the fire service was ten years well spent and above all I still miss the camaraderie. It's different with CrossFit. Camaraderie is very much part of the CrossFit ethos but when you're in a situation where people are in danger it tends to adopt a slightly different meaning. Sport can create great drama but one of the big plus points is that everyone usually goes home alive. Trust is therefore a prerequisite among firefighters – when you put your life in your team's hands on a daily basis, it naturally means you have a special bond with them. I think I still have that bond, in a way. Not only with individuals, but with the job itself. That said, ultimately leaving the fire service was not an easy decision to make, but it was the right one and I was hugely excited about the future.

CHAPTER 19:

IF YOU FALL OFF THE BIKE, GET BACK ON

In their ongoing quest to make the opening to the new CrossFit season more interesting, in 2014 CrossFit co-founder Greg Glassman, Games director Dave Castro and their team at CrossFit HQ decided to pitch several past champions against each other in the final announcement workout. To shake it up even more they decided to make it a mixed event and the athletes taking part were going to be Rich Froning, Jason Khalipa, Graham Holmberg, Annie Thorisdottir and me. With all five athletes lined up alongside each other it was obviously being staged as a big race and when I first got the call about it I was like, okay, good idea! We'd had a couple of mixed events at the CrossFit Games before such as a swim and a run but they'd never put us against each other in a CrossFit-style workout. This event was obviously going to be intense and, although there was no prize as such, there was an awful lot of pride at stake.

Because of our injuries, Annie and I hadn't competed against each other since she first won the Games, so for many people that was a big talking point. On a more personal front, Annie had won the CrossFit Games in both 2011 and 2012, so people always questioned whether, had she been there in 2013, she would have won again. The comments themselves were like water off a duck's back to me as you could probably generate hundreds of permutations as to who might have beaten who had they been fit. When all's said and done, Iceland Annie and I hadn't competed against each other for over three years so I was interested to see if she was back to her old formidable self, and if I was able to beat her.

The event took place in San Francisco and even I was surprised by the amount of interest the competition had generated. Then again, it was something that had never been done before and, with CrossFit growing globally, getting to watch a five-champions throwdown was manna from heaven for everyone.

The workout, '14.5', consisted of 21-18-15-12-9-6-3 reps, for time, of thrusters and burpees, and when Dave Castro told us to start I came out of the blocks very quickly indeed. I don't usually go out so hard but I wasn't sure how Annie was going to tackle the workout so I wanted to get out in front and see if she would push.

I felt good until the twelves and was fading into the nines when Rich Froning started to catch me up. I could see he was just a few seconds behind me. Because he was in the next lane, and because he's Rich Froning, I'd been aware of him from the start and as I gradually tired a feeling of inevitability began to sweep over me. Sure enough, about halfway through my set of nine reps, Mr Froning caught me up. I did have a bit of an internal battle at this point as half of me was saying, *Come on, catch him up*, whereas the other half was saying, *It doesn't matter. It's Rich Froning*. Although he didn't go firing off into the distance, Rich had a little bit more in the tank than I did so the second voice prevailed and I just kept my pace instead of trying to catch him back. Jokingly, I said to the commentator afterwards that I let him win! I don't think Rich had been listening when I said it so he was unaware and fortunately everyone seemed to take it in the right spirit. I did challenge him to a one-to-one during that interview but he never answered. He was obviously terrified. Understandably.

When I arrived in San Francisco I'd been lying first in the Open and, after putting in that performance, I ended up winning it by the largest-ever margin. I honestly don't think I'd ever felt fitter at this point and, without wanting to sound like a walking cliché machine, I felt I was on top of the world. I was also completely injury-free at the time so it's fair to say that the 2014 Regionals couldn't come quickly enough for me. Also, I knew that Annie would be stronger by then, and I was looking forward to having a proper head-to-head.

They say you should be careful what you wish for and me wishing for the Regionals to hurry up was, in hindsight, not a mistake exactly, but certainly foolhardy. In fact, looking back, I wish they'd never happened! Once again, the event took place in Copenhagen and on arrival I was still in excellent shape. To cut a long story short, the first events on day one were a max weight hang snatch into a max distance handstand walk (whoopee!) and basically I had an absolute nightmare on the walk. I took twenty-sixth place in that event. When I say I had a nightmare what I actually mean is that my best in that movement simply wasn't good enough and there were a lot of people in Europe who did a lot better than I did.

Going into day one I was actually more nervous about the hang snatch, but I managed to put up a competitive weight, tying for fifth place. So I was feeling happy and pumped going into the walk. I kicked up and felt pretty good; I didn't manage any record but I was still confident I'd done enough on the two workouts to be in a good position. Unfortunately, when I saw the leader board the reality of the situation set in. I tried to not think about it too much and focus on the job in hand. I went out hard on event three and, even though I took the win, I finished the first day out of contention of qualifying for the Games.

Giving up was never going to be an option but, even before my head hit the pillow that night, I knew it was going to be almost impossible to get back to third, which is where I had to be in order to qualify. Tenacity and determination notwithstanding, I still spent most of that night trying to come to terms with the fact that I probably wouldn't be defending my title and I'm not exaggerating when I say that it was probably one of the hardest and most counter-intuitive things I've ever had to do. Defending my title meant everything to me at the time and in that moment it felt like my life's work. I was also in a good place physically despite the handstand walk so everything felt wrong somehow.

Over the next two days we did four events and I fought like hell to get as far up the leader board as possible. It was going to be scant conciliation but if I was going to go out now I had to be completely satisfied that I'd done everything in my power to try to turn the situation around. Had I not, I'm not sure I could have lived with myself in that environment. In events four to six I did well, finishing second, first and first respectively. Going into the seventh and final workout, sixty-four pull-ups followed by eight overhead squats, I gave it everything I had, but during the overhead squats I saw Kristin Holte and Katrin Davidsdottir cross the finish line ahead of me. The weight seemed to double and when I saw Bjork Odinsdottir cross the line I knew my chance of qualifying was over and I failed the weight. Finding the motivation to finish the workout, knowing I wouldn't be returning to the Games, was one of the hardest things I've ever had to do. I had to fight back all the emotions to pick the bar back up and complete the remaining overhead squats, finishing the event in eighth and fourth overall on the leader board.

Looking back, my biggest frustration from this entire episode was denying myself the chance to compete at the highest level at what was probably my physical peak. It's one of those 'what if' scenarios, I suppose, and unfortunately I'll never know the outcome.

So many things were running through my head. What made the whole thing especially difficult was that, in previous years, past CrossFit champions wouldn't take a qualifying spot, so, had that rule still stood in 2014, I'd have qualified, and Oxana Slivenko too. There were other permutations that would have made a difference but they appeared in the following year. Either way, I hadn't qualified for the 2014 CrossFit Games and that was that. In terms of disappointment this was probably worse than pulling out through injury as at least then I actually wasn't fit enough to compete. The current CrossFit champion and fittest woman on earth messing up the handstand walk to such an extent that it denied her passage to the Games was not something I could easily live with at the time.

Despite the disappointment, the most important thing to me at the Regionals, other than qualifying for the Games, was acting like a champion and so even after I found out where I'd finished I kept a smile on my face, laughed and joked and encouraged the other athletes. At the end of the day it was no one's fault but my own and losing or failing is all part of sport. After all, if qualifying for the Games was easy, then I probably wouldn't want to still be fighting every year to get back. Sometimes you've just got to pull yourself together. And after the initial upset, life goes on and you learn from these experiences more than the winning. I think Katrin would agree with me here, as in the same Regionals she failed to qualify because of the rope climb workout. It's safe to say that in 2015 she came back a completely different athlete.

When you fall off your bike they say the best thing to do is get straight back on, so the day after the Regionals I found a gym in Copenhagen and did what I knew best and trained. I've never been one to feel sorry for myself and sure enough the heartache I'd experienced after not qualifying was already starting to ease off. Had I been an individual athlete, as in somebody who trained and competed primarily on their own, I dare say I'd have spent a few days licking my wounds with my coach or family but the fact is I wasn't. I was a CrossFit athlete and that meant something very different. With this in mind I decided to get on a plane and attend the Regionals that hadn't taken place yet. This might sound quite altruistic – you know, current CrossFit champion goes to lend her support – but the fact is that, despite not qualifying for the Games, I still wanted to be at the heart of CrossFit and the best way of doing that was to get off my bum, get to the remaining Regionals and encourage those who were still competing. Speaking selfishly, this was just what the doctor ordered. I did a lot of cheering, a lot of shouting, a lot of training, and when the final athletes had confirmed their places at the 2014 CrossFit Games my demons had been exorcised. Well, almost. Bloody handstand walks!

Because I'd been spending more and more time there, and because they still had the lion's share of CrossFit competitions (it's different now), in the summer of 2014 I decided to move out to America. The idea, apart from having some fun, was to compete in as many competitions as I possibly could. This was actually a necessity, as not competing in the CrossFit Games meant that I was going to be out of the loop for a while, or at least out of the top tier. In order to remain competitive and attractive to sponsors, I had to carry on competing so it ticked both boxes, personal and professional.

They might not have been as prestigious as the Games, but the events I competed in all featured at least a handful of current Games athletes and I managed to podium at just about every competition. It was actually a really good time for me, not just in terms of podiums, but in terms of getting to know new people. My training also improved as the CrossFit community over there was not only larger but a bit more advanced, and I was now working with three amazing coaches, Laura Phelps-Sweatt, Danny Lopez and Sean Lind.

At the risk of repeating myself – again – I went into 2015 feeling absolutely fantastic. Despite the Games, or lack of them, the second half of 2014 had been a success overall and, as well as feeling confident about the year to come, I was feeling strong.

You remember earlier when I said that having an injury is better than performing badly? Well, exactly one week before the 2015 Open my back went. We all assumed it was a recurring issue I'd had with my sacroiliac (SI) joint. I went to get treatment from a chiro and therapist and modified my training, which seemed to help. But it felt very unfair: at no point had I felt like I was overdoing it as there'd been no warning signs. In fact, my lifting numbers throughout the summer of 2014 had been brilliant. I was supposed to be at my peak, for heaven's sake! I was absolutely gutted. And I was in pain. Lots of pain.

The only thing I'd been suffering from at all since landing in America was plantar fasciitis, which causes pain around your heel and arch. It occurs when the fascia underneath your foot gets too tight and in my own experience it was always worse first thing in the morning. Sometimes it would feel like I'd broken my heel when I got out of bed. However, it hadn't really hindered me in any way as I'd only had to take running out of my training, which wasn't a huge worry. Apart from that I'd been A1 and my back in particular had been feeling really strong.

From a CrossFit point of view, the only thing I had going in my favour was that the Open was usually more about fitness than strength. So, depending on what the workouts were, there was a chance I could get through it. The reason they often concentrate on fitness over strength in the Open is to encourage mass participation, so, although I didn't know exactly what they were going to throw at us (nobody does!), I was confident there'd be no nasty surprises. As long as I used the seven days wisely and didn't do anything stupid, I was sure I'd be able to take part. I was so annoyed, though. How unlucky can you get?

Unfortunately, the God of totally inappropriate workouts had taken charge of the Open this year and, when I found out that the first workout of 2015 was going to be a max clean and jerk, I almost choked. It was just sod's law. Fortunately, you have five days to complete the workout from it being announced, which gave me five more days of rehab. It may not sound like much but I'd made progress in the week since sustaining the injury and, although I wouldn't be challenging for first position or anything, at least I'd be in with a chance of doing well.

While not wishing to sound arrogant, my ultimate aim at the Open had always been to finish among the top, whereas now it was simply to qualify for the Regionals. This shift in mentality was instinctive and when I finally did the first workout you could say I was in full-on survival mode. The workout was in two parts – the first involved doing as many reps as possible in 9 minutes of 15 toes-to-bar, ten deadlifts and five snatches, both at 34kg. It was the first time I'd had to wear a belt for deadlifts so light! The second part was hitting a maximum clean and jerk in 6 minutes. I knew I had to give everything on the first part as the clean and jerk was going to be pretty impossible for me to put up a competitive score. Warming up I couldn't even lift 70kg. But I gave myself a serious self-talk and attacked the workout. For the first part I got the second-best score in the world – which went some way to salvaging my lift, where I came a slightly less impressive 1,511th. But I was as happy as I could be in the circumstances: I had managed to lift 84kg which was a miracle given the state of my back. Most importantly, I was still in with a chance of qualifying for the Regionals.

After week one I had a cortisone injection to help alleviate the pain, which helped my back to hold out throughout the rest of the competition. It's just as well I did, as the live announcement for week five was going to feature the last three female winners of the CrossFit Games – Camille Leblanc-Bazinet, me and Annie Thorisdottir. I was a tiny bit daunted by this prospect, but not nearly as daunted as I was excited. I said earlier that nothing pushes you like strong competition. Well, these two girls were two of the strongest on earth at the time and, when I set off to Vegas to take part in the announcement, all thoughts of SI joints and plantar fasciitis disappeared. Saying that, this was going to take a big, big effort, and I had no idea if I was up to it. I hoped I was.

The workout itself was, for time, a 27-21-15-9 couplet of calories rowed and thrusters. It was a big shock to the crowd as it was the first time CrossFit hadn't included a form of burpees in the Open.

As expected, all three of us went unbroken on the thrusters so it really came down to how fast each of us could row. By the third round I'd managed to pull away from Annie, and Camille, who was leading the Open worldwide at the time, was back in third. This was going well! I hadn't felt a twinge from my back so as far as I was concerned I was cured. Or was I?

When I sat down for my final row, Annie was too far behind to catch me and I managed to win with a time of 7 minutes flat. What's really inspiring about taking part in an event like that is that around 300,000 people around the world are going to be doing exactly the same workout over the next week. You're helping to start something quite amazing really.

By winning the workout I'd done enough to qualify for the Regionals (I finished eighty-second overall) and I genuinely felt like I was back to my old self again. Or I was at least getting there. The following day, however, I went to the gym as normal. I was doing squat cleans, building up the weight and everything was feeling great, but then as I went to stand one up it was like someone had run at me with a baseball bat and everything went into spasm.

I knew instinctively what had happened. I felt I'd let my back heal up, but it had obviously just held together during the Open and now it was going on strike. My body was saying, *Okay, Sam, I've got you through the Open. Now you have to let me rest and heal properly.* I couldn't have argued even if I'd wanted to. I was a bit disappointed but in truth I wasn't really surprised. The rehab had been papering over a crack and the crack now needed filling.

When I got back to Miami from Vegas I went straight in for an MRI scan to see what the damage was. It was more serious than the suspected SI joint injury: I had two bulging discs and a herniated one in my back. After I took the results to a specialist we we started working out how I was going to get fixed. With the Regionals just over a month away, the rehab had to be intensive but at the same time it had to be thorough. Despite what you've just read, I do usually listen to my body; with my back I knew it wasn't something I could just work through. I would have to be sensible with rehab and training in order to be able to compete at the Regionals. After modifying my training (again!), I got to work and by the first week of May everything seemed to be good. I obviously wasn't back up to 100 per cent but working with a specialist I was able to get my back to the point I'd be able to compete at the Regionals, providing I didn't do anything silly, of course, like go and injure myself beforehand.

CHAPTER 20:

PUTTING MY FOOT IN IT

Exactly one week before the 2015 Atlantic Regional was due to take place I broke my foot. Yes, I'm afraid you read that correctly. I broke my foot. I was living in Miami at the time, and after getting out of bed that morning I realised very quickly that I couldn't put any weight at all on my right foot. In fact, it was incredibly painful and I remember swearing quite a bit. What the hell was up with me now? I wondered. I waited to see if the pain would die down but it didn't, so after using my left leg to compensate I finally managed to get myself out of bed.

There wasn't much swelling at all and I'd not done anything crazy the day before or felt anything in training so I decided to just try to walk it off. This might sound slightly ridiculous to some people but having suffered from plantar fasciitis I knew that sometimes this did the trick. Time's a great healer, or so they say. It really felt like I'd just sprained something, but I'd never felt a sensation like that before. I went into the gym as usual and mentioned it to my coach, who suggested that as I was going for treatment that day I should mention it while I was there. When I hobbled into the therapist's office, she said, 'Just the usual?' and, almost forgetting about the foot, I replied, 'Yes please.' But then as I got up onto the treatment bed the pain reminded me that I should say something about my foot.

'It's probably nothing,' I assured her. 'I've probably just sprained it or something, but could you just have a look to make sure?'

Thank you, Dr Briggs!

Fortunately, the therapist had received a tad more medical training than I had and after taking one look at my foot she said, 'We'll get an x-ray just to be safe.' I tried persuading her that it wasn't needed but she was adamant. Even then I assumed this was just a precautionary measure and, after she returned with the results, I was expecting her to endorse my own course of treatment which I confidently predicted would be painkillers and rest. Well, painkillers. I'm not very good at rest.

The therapist had other ideas. 'I'm afraid you need to go and see our podiatrist,' she said. 'We've got your results and she's in at the moment so she'd like to see you.'

I was still thinking this was overkill. I really just wanted to get back to the gym and train. But when I walked into the podiatrist's office she told me to sit down immediately and then I knew there was something wrong.

'I can't believe you just walked yourself in here!' she said. 'The pain must be incredible.'

Still trying to brush the severity off I protested, 'It just feels sprained.'

'It's more than that, I'm afraid. You have what's sometimes known as a dancer's fracture,' said the podiatrist.

I was about to say something like, *I don't dance*, but I thought better of it.

'Its correct name is a fifth metatarsal avulsion fracture,' she continued.

After further explanation, it appeared the fracture was close to a tendon. These are easily displaced and the reason she'd been so alarmed was because I shouldn't have been walking on it for a minute, let alone most of the day.

'You'll need a boot and crutches immediately,' ordered the podiatrist.

'But how long for?' I asked.

'Oh, at least six weeks. Could be more like eight or nine, though.'

'But I've got the Regionals in a week,' I said in a panic.

'No chance,' countered the podiatrist. 'I'm afraid you need to rest it, Sam.'

After being issued with a fracture foot boot and two crutches, I left the clinic and went straight to the gym, hoping to find my coach. Fortunately, he was there. When he saw me hobble in on crutches and with a foot boot on, his chin almost hit the floor.

'Oh my God, Sam,' he said. 'I wasn't expecting this.'

'Neither was I,' I replied. 'It's a bit of a mess, isn't it?'

After he ushered me through to the office area, I told my coach exactly what the podiatrist had said. He was obviously as shocked as I was and, as he asked what I was going to do, I could only reply with a shrug and 'I don't know'. As I sat there in the office I could feel myself going into full-on misery mode. I'd had this feeling before, and I didn't like it.

Ten minutes later I was back in the gym training. My coach wasn't happy about it but he knew what I was like so he didn't say anything. I'd missed the Games in 2014 and had managed to get through the 2015 Open with one herniated disc and two bulging ones. There was absolutely no way I was giving up now. Boot or no boot, I was giving it a go.

Just as an aside, I would not recommend this course of action to anybody else. If you're sitting at home with a foot boot on after being told to rest up and let your injury heal, please do exactly that!

The catalyst for me removing the boot and hobbling into the gym was a notion that this could be my last year competing. Yes, that old chestnut. As soon as that occurred to me I felt an overwhelming compulsion to get up and train and who am I to argue with an overwhelming compulsion? This was obviously a similar thought pattern to the one I'd had when I'd turned thirty about not being able to win the CrossFit Games if I was older. The goal had been downgraded slightly, but the compulsion had been the same. In fact, if anything the desire to carry on training now was probably stronger than before, as the alternative was more final. Competing and training were everything to me.

It was all very well me claiming I was going to train and compete with a broken foot, but in order to be able to continue doing so I had to ask some massive favours. They're far too numerous to mention here but one of the most important was when Talayna Fortunato, who is also a therapist, drove a four-hour round trip to try out different taping techniques that would help move any weight I was carrying to the other side of the foot and away from the fracture. What makes this gesture really special is that the day she drove over was her mother's birthday and because they were spending the day together her mother came too. I felt awful when I found out but the help she gave me was invaluable. It doesn't stop there, though. Talayna had stopped competing by this time and after teaching me how to tape my foot she offered to fly out to the Regionals with me and act as my therapist. She'd be able to tape the foot up before each event and then provide treatment after to minimise any pain and discomfort I was in.

The only slight worry I had prior to the Regionals was me potentially being barred by the organisers on medical grounds. I had to keep my injury a secret, otherwise I wouldn't have been allowed to compete. Incidentally, because I was now living in Miami, I had to switch from competing at the European Regional to the Atlantic Regional, which covers the east coast of America. So this would be my first year competing in a new region, trying to hide the fact I had a broken foot. Under new changes announced at the 2014 CrossFit Invitational, regions were now combined into super-regions (the Atlantic was now the combined Mid Atlantic and South West regions) with only five athletes qualifying for the Games. This made the Regionals even more competitive.

The first workout at this year's Regionals, called 'Randy', comprised of seventy-five snatches with 55lb/25kg and my strategy in this workout was to go unbroken. The field was obviously strong and with it being the first event of a new region I wanted to start well, especially because I knew this was one I could push hard without hurting my foot too much. Fortunately, I was able to back up my ambition and managed to complete the workout in 2 minutes 28 seconds. Cassidy Lance was the next athlete over the line with a 2:45 followed by Anna Tunnicliffe with a 2:52. I surprised myself in the second workout, a chipper featuring thrusters and rope climbs, by finishing second behind Anna, and so I finished day one with a big smile on my face. My foot wasn't smiling, but that was just tough.

The first workout on day two was another chipper and it started off with a 1-mile/1.6km run on a TrueForm Runner – a kind of self-propelled treadmill. I hadn't been looking forward to this one little bit as I had never used one of these runners before and with my foot in its current state I wasn't going to be able to practise before the event. But, as with workout number one, I had a strategy. It was quite similar to that one really – go as fast as you bloody can so you can get off the thing – and when I stepped off the treadmill first I was absolutely thrilled to bits. When people found out about the injury, they all asked me how I was able to run so quickly but that was an easy question to answer.

'It hurt like hell so I had to get it done as quickly as possible!'

In the same workout we had to do 150 double-unders and 100 box jump overs which I was also looking forward to – not! I had to do the double-unders on one leg and instead of jumping up and jumping down on two legs for the box jump overs I would jump up and then step down carefully. Mum told me afterwards that this is where the commentators started catching onto the fact that I was carrying an injury.

By the end of the workout I was in a tie for first place overall and had managed to build up a buffer between first and sixth place of about 80 points. When I tell you what the next event was you'll realise how important that buffer was going to be. That's right, it was the dreaded handstand walk. My nemesis! Although it didn't affect my foot, it had obviously been my downfall at the previous year's Regional and I was desperate for it not to be my downfall here. We had to cover a distance of 250 feet/76 metres in 3 minutes and unfortunately I missed out by a few metres, which was at least good enough for fourteenth, a big improvement from twenty-sixth. After finishing the max weight snatch in eleventh position, I was able to take second and fifth on the last day's events, finishing the 2015 Atlantic Regional competition in second position overall.

I know it sounds slightly cliched, but because of all the permutations surrounding my foot I really did have to take this competition one workout at a time, both physically and mentally. It was an essential part of me qualifying for the 2015 CrossFit Games.

The day after the competition, I flew out to Los Angeles to see a surgeon. One of my sponsors, Progenex's Paul Gomez, had contacts with Red Bull and he'd very kindly arranged an appointment with one of the surgeons who looked after their athletes. Because Red Bull sponsor so many extreme sports, their athletes tend to follow suit in terms of injuries and so their surgeons were obviously used to seeing all kinds of horrendous things, often far worse than mine. Most importantly, they understood the importance of getting an athlete on their feet again as soon as possible. That, primarily, is why I was so keen on accepting the appointment.

I'd already been told that if the bone had been displaced by more than 10 per cent I'd have to have surgery which would require me to have pins in my foot. Regardless of how proficient the Red Bull surgeons were, that was going to keep me out for a long time. Most alarmingly, it was going to keep me out of the Games.

It was a pretty nerve-wracking time waiting for the results of that consultation. Even I wouldn't be able to compete with a pot on my lower leg and pins in my feet. Then again, I'd probably give it a go.

When the surgeon came back, he said that fortunately the bone had only been displaced by 5 per cent so, providing I was careful with it and wore a boot for the next six weeks, he wouldn't have to operate. What a relief! I'd obviously have to modify my training somewhat again and after four weeks I'd have a check-up to make sure everything was okay. I wasn't actually out of the woods at this point as there was still a chance it might not have healed quickly enough. Thankfully, I had nothing to worry about and for the two weeks leading up to the Games I was able to ditch the boot and start training somewhat normally. I still had to put the boot back on between sessions but this was the closest I'd come to training conventionally in many months and it couldn't have come at a better time.

The only other change at this point was a move to California. The sponsor who put me in touch with Red Bull had very kindly offered me an apartment in LA and with the Games just around the corner I accepted the offer. California was more central to my activities and, with the Games taking place there, it was perfect place to train in the run-up. I also had a lot of friends living in California so all things considered it was a very welcome opportunity.

My mindset going into the 2015 CrossFit Games was dominated by gratitude. Ultra-competitive athlete or not, I couldn't get beyond the fact that I shouldn't really have been there. Anything here on in was going to be a bonus and my sole ambition was to enjoy the experience as much as I possibly could. I hadn't excluded myself from trying, of course. Anything but. I've said many times that giving my all is a prerequisite with me, whatever I'm doing. This wasn't going to be any different. But, still feeling far from as strong as I needed to be, I knew the odds were stacked against me if I wanted to make an impression at these Games ...

CHAPTER 21:

PEDAL TO THE METAL

For the fourth year in a row, the 2015 CrossFit Games started on a Wednesday and being able to travel to them by car instead of plane and not three weeks beforehand was bliss. One of the biggest advantages of moving to California was climatisation. The temperatures in California that year were almost off the scale, so one of the biggest challenges facing the athletes was going to be heat exhaustion.

Fortunately for all concerned, the first event of the 2015 CrossFit Games took place in the Pacific Ocean and consisted of two 500-metre swims with a 2-mile/3.2km paddle on a prone paddle board sandwiched in between. When CrossFit athletes are called to the water, we either thrive or flounder but, with the addition of a paddle board this year, things were going to be harder to predict. As most athletes had never used the prone boards before, it was going to be chaos. The Aussies were like racing pros up on their knees taking huge powerful strokes, gliding across the water. Everyone else, me included, was lying flat, glued to the board and fearing for our lives! I had a severely chafed chin but managed to finish seventh, which I was really happy with.

Once we'd all dried off, it was back to the StubHub Center in Carson to compete in a sandbag move, which had last been seen at the CrossFit Games back in 2010. That year, we'd had to transport sandbags weighing a total of 370lb/168kg from the top of some stairs on one side of the stadium to the top of the stairs at the other, using a basic wheelbarrow from a hardware store. This year, Rogue had designed a set of 250lb/113kg wheelbarrows and the organisers had upped the weight to, in total, 480lb/218kg. I was actually one of only six finalists who'd done this workout before but that held no advantage. Despite coming second in my heat behind Annie, I tied tenth for the workout. This left me in fifth place overall at the end of day one and, given everything I'd been through before the Games, I'd take it.

Thursday was a rest day but on the Friday we came crashing back to earth with a bump when the organisers instructed us to strap on a 14lb/6kg weight vest each and tackle a workout called 'Murph'. Murph is named after a CrossFit hero called Mike Murphy, or Navy Lieutenant Michael Murphy, to give him his full title. Mike was tragically killed in Afghanistan on 28 June 2005 and was posthumously awarded the Congressional Medal of Honour. The workout was one of his favourites and apparently he used to call it Body Armour because of the weighted vests. Whenever CrossFitters tackle Murph, we always do so in remembrance of Mike and it's become a tradition in America to perform the workout on Memorial Day.

While the average CrossFitter might decide to break up the 100 pull-ups, 200 push-ups and 300 air squats that make up the three parts of this workout, we had to perform them in order, meaning that we couldn't move on to the next movement until we'd completed all the reps of the previous one. Add in a 1-mile/1.6km run either side of these movements and you have the makings of a potentially devastating challenge.

On day one the heat had been blistering in California but on the Friday it was almost unbearable. It must have been at least forty degrees centigrade. After everyone decided to sprint the first 100 metres of the mile run, I managed to start picking people off and, although Anna Tunnicliffe was the first woman to return to the stadium, Kristin Holte, Alethea Boon and I weren't far behind her. Then by the time we got to the press-ups I was neck and neck with Alethea at the front of the field. The air squats seemed to last forever but this is where I managed to create a gap between me and the rest of the field. The difference between how I moved during the first run and how I moved during the second is enormous, and if I were to explain it in terms of age I look like a 33-year-old athlete in the first run and a 95-year-old athlete in the second. To be fair, that's about how old I felt leaving the stadium on run two. However, looking back at the footage, Alethea Boon runs exactly the same in the second race as she did in the first. It's actually quite scary! I think my lead was about 45 seconds at the start of run two and fortunately as time went on my body started loosening up a bit.

I only heard this afterwards, but one of the commentators said during the second run that I'd probably entered more competitions in the off-season than any other female athlete in the sport. Whether that was true or not I honestly couldn't tell you but it didn't surprise me – I'd gone on a mission after not making the Games in 2014 and entered almost every other big competition out there, which had ultimately resulted in my back injury. It was another reminder that perhaps I should take it a little easier in the off-season, not that that would ever be easy for me.

Something else the commentator made reference to was that, when I came into the stadium to complete my second run, the clock was at 38.5 minutes and during the men's event some athletes had still been doing air squats prior to their second run at 55 minutes. I just thought I'd mention it. We're entitled to a bit of girl power every now and then.

To be honest, the last quarter of a mile or so was actually okay and the reception I received running into the stadium, which was very noisy indeed, enabled me to move into something resembling a sprint. Well, loosely. I finished in a time of 39 minutes 10 seconds and, had I been competing in the men's event, that would have put me second. Sorry, more girl power!

Because of the extreme heat and humidity, eight men and four women failed to complete the event and Kara Saunders had to be given treatment for heatstroke after collapsing on the finish line. Kara managed to battle on and complete the competition, but others weren't as lucky and some like Annie Thorisdottir had to withdraw from the Games entirely after this workout, citing overheating and severe dehydration. I've seen the footage and her legs literally stop working halfway through the second run. It's quite upsetting to watch.

Whether or not it was my exertions in Murph that made the difference I'm not sure, but in workout number four, a snatch ladder, I ended up finishing in thirty-fifth position, so my day had literally gone from the sublime to the ridiculous. But, as I'm not known for my strength and had only been able to start lifting two weeks earlier, a thirty-fifth position was probably where I should have been!

The concluding workout on the Friday was another hero workout, i.e. one that's named after fallen servicemen and women. In this case it was 'DT', which is named in honour of Air Force Staff Sergeant Timothy P. Davis, who was killed by an IED in Afghanistan in February 2009. As with many CrossFit workouts, this actually looks quite harmless on paper but in practice it's anything but. It consists of five rounds for time of twelve deadlifts, nine hang power cleans and six push jerks and, announcing it earlier in the afternoon, Dave Castro had said there'd be a twist. Obviously this twist wasn't going to make it easier so when he imparted the details we were all ears. He said that the fans in attendance and the entire affiliate community watching the Games online and on ESPN would have the option to decide whether the competitors would perform 'Double DT', which is ten rounds instead of five, or 'Heavy DT', which for women is 145lb/66kg instead of 105lb/48kg. The votes were counted and the clear winner was, surprise surprise, Heavy DT. I don't know what that says about the CrossFit community!

Again, to demonstrate the sheer futility of form books at this competition, Tia-Clair Toomey, who was currently lying fourth and would finish second overall, finished this event in thirty-first position and had finished Murph in twenty-seventh. Forgone conclusions are extremely rare in CrossFit but this was taking the unpredictability to a different level. Incidentally, I ended up finishing fifteenth in this one so if you discount the disastrous snatch speed ladder I was doing okay.

In the eight remaining workouts I needed at least a couple of firsts, and maybe a second to get anywhere near the podium.

Fortunately, in the last workout of the Saturday I managed to get a second which, from my point of view, was going to make day four very interesting indeed. The workout in question was a triangle couplet (15-10-6 thrusters and bar muscle-ups). The common CrossFit thruster weight for females would be 95lb/43kg but, this being the Games, they raised the stakes to 115lb/52kg. Camille Leblanc-Bazinet ruled this workout by finishing in a soaring 4:47 in an earlier heat, some 45 seconds before me. But not knowing her time I gave it my all and was happy to win my heat and finish second behind her. My foot, by the way, had been behaving itself but the lack of training I'd been able to do beforehand had definitely hindered me on the heavier events. That was always going to be inevitable so shifting my mindset and restricting my ambitions had been a very good idea. In competition it's pointless getting frustrated by things that are out of your control. I had done the best I could to prepare myself for the Games, so I could only do as well as I could. Concentrating on each workout in hand and just doing my absolute best meant that I was happy and enjoying the experience regardless of my position on the leader board. That being said, I was still aiming to climb it!

Despite my efforts in the couplet, I was still lying outside the top ten so, if I was going to get anywhere near the podium, I was going to have to produce something special on the final day. A top ten place certainly wasn't beyond me and for all the talk of restricting my ambitions I'd be lying if I said I wasn't longing to smash the final workouts and make it onto the podium. Of course I was.

The first workout of the final day was announced as six rounds of a 400-metre run including one steep incline followed by a 50-foot/15-metre yoke carry with 300lb/136kg. Providing my foot held out, I was confident of doing well in this workout and, sure enough, I managed to put in an above-average performance. I'm underplaying this slightly as I actually finished first and this moved me all the way up to sixth position on the leader board. With two workouts to go I had a small chance of making it onto the podium. It was going to take a miracle, of course, but being in that position so close to the finish was seriously intoxicating. I was ready to give everything I had.

The two final workouts, entitled Pedal to the Metal 1 and 2, consisted of the following movements. PTTM1 had three pegboard ascents (climbing up a vertical board using movable pegs and upper-body strength alone), a 24-calorie row, a 16-calorie bike sprint and eight dumbbell squat snatches to be completed in a time of 6 minutes. PTTM2 had twelve parallette handstand push-ups, a 24-calorie row, a 16-calorie bike sprint and eight kettlebell deadlifts to be completed in a time of 7 minutes.

Regardless of what was going to happen to me, there were several athletes, male and female, who were in genuine contention for the title at this point so it had all the makings of being a classic. This was notched up another gear when the first three places in PTTM1 were taken by athletes sitting outside the top ten. The pegboard, which I don't think any of us had ever seen before, let alone tackled, turned out to be everyone's worst nightmare, and with it being the first movement it shook everyone up a bit. The accumulated fatigue from the previous events meant that, try as we might, everyone was failing reps left, right and centre. The only athlete I could see who was practically flying up the pegboard was Margaux Alvarez. I watched carefully, trying to figure out what magical technique she was using, but it was no use. Even my nickname, 'Biceps Like Briggs', was failing me now as time after time I'd start the climb only for my arms to give way!

Unfortunately, I ended up finishing thirteenth in the workout, which meant the only way I could podium now was if I won the final event and everyone else around me had a shocker. There was nothing else for it then. I'd just have to put the pedal to the metal.

I actually led for most of the workout, until Katrin Davidsdottir, who wasn't known for her deadlifts, went unbroken on the deadlifts. I told you she came back a different athlete. She'd been in brilliant form throughout the competition and going unbroken was just a little bit beyond me. Katrin finished the workout in a time of 4:42 and I hit the finish mat, literally, about 9 seconds after her. Despite Katrin's heroics, Sara Sigmundsdottir had been clear favourite to win the title as she had a commanding lead going into the workout, so no one knew who'd won until Dave Castro made the announcement!

The final top ten for the 2015 CrossFit Games looked like this:

1st – Katrin Davidsdottir
2nd – Tia-Clair Toomey
3rd – Sara Sigmundsdottir
4th – Me
5th – Kara Saunders
6th – Chyna Cho
7th – Lindsey Valenzuela
8th – Emily Abbott
9th – Margaux Alvarez
10th – Amanda Goodman

Considering the year I'd had with injuries, I was over the moon with fourth. There were so many times I didn't think I'd even be on that competition floor so I certainly left the Games with quite a big smile on my face. Not a smug one. A grateful one. Part of me couldn't help wondering what might have happened had I been fully fit, but this was no time for what ifs. I'd just finished fourth fittest on earth, for heaven's sake!

CHAPTER 22:

A ONE-ARMED VISA-LESS ATHLETE

After the Games, disaster struck, and this time it wasn't an injury. I had gone to spend a few months in Cincinnati with a friend as a new relationship was blooming, and to work with Laura Phelps-Sweatt once again. During this time I was trying to apply for a green card to stay in the States; the initial application had been granted just before the Games. As I was filling in the paperwork, I began to suspect there was something wrong with the initial application. On recommendation from Camille – who'd just successfully obtained her card – I contacted her lawyer for advice. My fears were confirmed. The lawyer who had been advising me and who had completed my initial application had told me I had to remain in the USA while it was going through. He hadn't adjusted my status and, as I'd been there on a travel visa (ESTA), I had technically been in the USA longer than the ESTA allowance.

In order to get this sorted I went back to the United Kingdom and straight to the American Embassy but, despite my application for a green card being successful, I was now classed as an overstay. As a consequence, instead of staying and settling in the USA on a semi-permanent basis and continuing my CrossFit dream as I'd been hoping, I was banned from entering the country for three years. The ironic thing is that, had I stayed in the USA, it would probably have been sorted out earlier but I was trying to show I wasn't intentionally breaking the rules and trying to do things right.

This didn't just affect me professionally; it affected me personally too. I was now in a serious relationship with a fellow athlete, Nicole Holcomb, and me having to move back to the UK was not in our plans! I won't bore you with all the details but it's taken me, Nicole and several lawyers four long years and thousands of dollars to sort this out and I've only recently received my green card. Four years! Also, despite being in a relationship and getting married in that time, I wasn't even able to visit Nicole once in the USA. Nicole had a serious back injury so her flying to the UK on a regular basis was out of the question. In order to make the relationship work we had to spend our times together in Canada or we'd take trips to our friends in the Caymans. Long-distance relationships are not ideal but we made the best of what we could. Thank goodness for FaceTime!

I realise rules are rules, but I wasn't intentionally breaking them and had all the evidence to show that I was under the misguidance of a US attorney! Luckily, because of this fact, I was able to get special dispensation to still be able to compete at the CrossFit Games. But I wasn't able to compete in any other competitions in the USA, and most of the time it was a last-minute allowance, meaning a lot of stressful Games prep.

The end of 2015 was bittersweet to say the least. From a CrossFit point of view I'd surpassed all expectations and, because of how complicated everything had been with all the injuries, I was as proud as I'd ever been. The only silver lining from a personal point of view was that I was able to see my family and friends a lot more often than I had recently so it wasn't all doom and gloom. In fact, that was actually a big bonus and it prevented me from getting too down. Thank God I didn't know it would take four years to sort the green card issue out. My philosophical attitude may have changed slightly.

To take my mind off the green card woes, in January 2016, just over six years after first entering the British Indoor Rowing Championships back in November 2009 – when I'd become the British lightweight champion – I decided to enter it again. I'll be honest: a friend of mine talked me into it, and I initially wasn't keen. But, instead of being held at the Birmingham NEC like it had been before, it was being held in Manchester at the Velodrome and with every excuse I could think of not to go being used up I relented and said yes, signing up right at the last minute.

At the championships, you can enter one or two of the race events: a 2-kilometre row in the morning and a 500-metre row in the afternoon. I had signed up for both. By the time I reached the Velodrome, which is a really impressive venue, I was actually looking forward to it.

The first event went well, and I ended up setting a new British lightweight record in the 30–39 category with a time of 7:05.1. Not bad for a last-minute entry! However, after the 2km row – and anyone who has tried it will agree with me – I was absolutely smoked. My legs didn't feel my own, my lungs were bleeding and, after not eating much that morning to make weight, I was absolutely starving.

There were a few hours between events so I drove back into the centre of Manchester to my friend's house for some lunch. As I was now nicely fed and relaxed the last thing I wanted to do was go and give 100 per cent effort again on the same rower that had left me in so much pain that morning. But my friend, Chloe Barrett, was having none of it, and when I told her that I was thinking of doing a disappearing act she basically read me the riot act.

'It's 500 metres, for heaven's sake! Two minutes' work. Look, just sort yourself out and get it done. You'll feel better once you've done it!'

I'm afraid I was out-argued so, with my reputation still intact, just, I picked myself up, dusted myself down and prepared to start all over again. By the time it was my turn to row I actually felt quite good and, when the signal went to go, I set off like a bullet. This was a massive mistake as after just a few seconds I knew that exhaustion wasn't far away. What made it worse was that the time I was setting was very fast so I was left with two choices: give in to the tiredness and let inertia take over or dig in and fight for what could be another record. Somehow I managed to summon up the energy to do the latter and, instead of breaking the British record again, I ended up breaking the world record. The existing world record had been 1:36.7 and I'd smashed it by posting a time of 1:33.4. The thing is, I'd also smashed myself. To pieces! There's a video somewhere on YouTube of me directly after this row and I'm face down on the floor groaning. I was there for about ten minutes. I just couldn't move.

None of my records still stands, although I did manage to re-break my record while actually having some rowing training from Cameron Nichol, but unfortunately we never made it official. Indoor rowing is a sport in its own right and I'm sure they take their training seriously. So when a non-rower breaks a record they like to fight for it back! Although getting into a battle trying to break the record back could have been fun, I had my 2016 season to start preparing for: the CrossFit Open was now back in my sights and

I needed to concentrate on that. And there were already enough newcomers coming up through the ranks in CrossFit to keep me on my toes.

The interesting thing about the 2016 CrossFit Open, apart from me taking part without an injury, was that it hailed the dominance of a young athlete called Jamie Greene. Jamie's about ten years younger than I am (who isn't?) but one thing we have in common is that we both played rugby league. She trained as a gymnast though, so that's where the similarities stop really. In 2015, Jamie had finished 102nd overall in the Open. Then, at the 2016 Open she finished first overall, surprising everybody. What an announcement! I finished second, which wasn't too shoddy, but I remember thinking to myself when the final leader board was finalised, *This girl is going to be dangerous at the Regionals.*

Luckily for us, Jamie had already committed herself to competing with her team CrossFit YAS at the Regionals with the intention of making it to the Games in 2016. This meant we would have to wait until 2017 to see how dangerous as an individual she was going to be. Dangerous she has been: after finishing eighth in her debut year 2017 and eleventh after shoulder surgery in 2018, she got her first podium in 2019 by finishing third. It's always cool to see new athletes come into the sport who show potential, grow and make it into the upper echelons of CrossFit. It forces everyone's game up a bit. Once again, nothing motivates an athlete like strong competition and, when the athlete in question is ten years younger than you are and is obviously very talented, you've got two choices: give up or fight for your place. I'll always choose to try to fight for my place but it was also a stark reminder that I was fast becoming the grandma of CrossFit.

Speaking of being the grand old lady of CrossFit, shortly before the 2016 Regionals, my first back in Europe, I was invited to go and train with Sara Sigmundsdottir and a young Swiss athlete called Adrian Mundwiler. Adrian had only recently come onto the scene and he'd finished forty-second overall in this year's Open. He was also just twenty-four years of age, the same age as Sara.

On the first night at the training camp, Sara and Adrian stayed up watching reruns of *Friends* (something I've noticed a lot of Europeans are obsessed with watching), and thinking nothing of it I stayed up too and joined in the banter. But as the days went by, I was seriously starting to struggle with the training and couldn't for the life of me figure out why. Was I just getting too old to keep up? Then it struck me like a eureka moment. I'm not twenty-four; I need more sleep than these whippersnappers! So that night when they started to unwind with Phoebe and Joey, I bowed out as gracefully as I could and after hobbling out of the way I went upstairs, took out my false teeth and fell blissfully asleep.

The first event at the 2016 European Regional was a snatch workout and with this not being my strongest suit I'd trained hard for it. This, I suppose, was partly down to what had happened in 2014 with the dreaded handstand walk. That still played on my mind occasionally and with no injuries to take my mind off it (where are the broken feet when you need them?), I let nerves get the better of me. Instead of using them to fuel my performance I let negativity hinder me. I knew I wasn't going to win this event but I did far worse than I had in practice, finishing in twenty-fifth position.

The next event was 'Nate'; I managed to fare a little better, taking seventh, but it wasn't enough to pull me into the top ten at the end of day one. This meant that for the start of day two I was in a different heat to Sara, Annie and Kristin Holte. I had to go before them and hope I could post a competitive time to try to climb back into a qualifying spot. I couldn't judge my performance on those around me so I was basically racing myself. This was an awful situation to be in. But I knew how to fight and I wanted to be back at the Games, so fight was what I was going to do!

Taking a third, first and second on day two saw me back in the top heat for the final day where an eighth and first saw me finishing fourth overall in the competition behind Sara, Annie and Kristin. The final workout was actually an epic sprint finish between me, Annie and Sara with just a hundredth of a second separating us, definitely worth a YouTube view!

Fourth place in 2014 as you'll remember wouldn't have qualified me for the Games, but with Europe and the Meridian region having merged to make super-regions, the top five athletes from a more competitive field would qualify. It's hard to describe the relief I felt when I found out I'd made it but I didn't let on. No way. I was as cool as a cucumber. Well, I do have a huge smile on all the photos but I always smile, right?!

How long is it since I had an injury? A few pages? Well, about a month before the 2016 CrossFit Games were due to take place, I began struggling with my shoulder. It started off as just a twinge but within a few days I was unable to move my left arm more than a couple of inches from my body. I remember walking around the gym in a state of complete denial – again – looking for something to train on that only required one arm, when Craig Massey, one of the head coaches and business partners, came up to me and asked if I was okay. This, I'm afraid, was a catalyst for me losing the plot a bit and, as the tears began to appear, I heard myself saying to him,

'Not only can I not go to the Games because of my visa problem, now I can't even train!'

'Why not?' he asked.

'I can't move my arm.'

'Really?'

'Really.'

'Oh dear [it may have been a stronger word here]. That's not good.'

'You're telling me.'

The first person I contacted when it all went wrong was James Jowsey, my former movement mechanics coach. We'd drifted apart since I moved to the USA but I knew he'd be able to help. Sure enough, he knew exactly what we needed to do in the short term. And so, with literally a week to spare, James and I got to work on making my arm move again. It was the strangest feeling, not having the use of it. Also, the fact that it wasn't that painful actually made it worse as I had nothing really to blame it on. It was as if my arm had been possessed by somebody. Somebody very lazy! This was all just a temporary measure, by the way. Something to get me through the Games. I'd get it seen to properly afterwards.

While all this was going on I was trying to sort out my visa, and with less than a week to go I still hadn't been given clearance by the American Embassy. In a last-ditch attempt to get some help I reached out to my Instagram followers to see if anyone could help me. That's how desperate the situation was. I was a one-armed, visa-less athlete trying to get to America to compete to be the fittest woman on earth and I was having to turn to social media to get there. The reaction from the CrossFit community was, unsurprisingly, tremendous and with the help of a few contacts we chased up leads and had many telephone calls, until finally we managed to get special dispensation, with hours to spare. Well, at least it took my mind off my arm and shoulder.

Speaking of which.

Luckily for me, James Jowsey was also attending the Games with a team called CrossFit Yas, who had Jamie Greene in their ranks. He was helping them out so, hopefully, if he had time, he'd be able to help me out too.

By the time I landed at San Diego airport I was mentally and physically exhausted. Preparation-wise, in the weeks leading up to the Games, I'd spent the majority of my time working with James on my arm or pleading to anyone who'd listen about getting to LA, while still trying to train full-time on the off-chance that I actually made it there. There was also an eight-hour time difference between the UK and California so I knew that jetlag wouldn't be far away. With my nerves also in a bit of a state it was anyone's guess how I'd get on. Then again, the website barbend.com, who'd reported on my visa issues, had said, and I quote: 'A jetlagged Sam Briggs is still a pretty damn scary Sam Briggs.' Scary, me? They obviously meant that I was down but not out. I'm not scary, am I?

Whatever happened, *philosophical statement warning*, it was definitely going to be character-building.

CHAPTER 23:

TIME TO
RE-EVALUATE

The thing I needed most at the start of the 2016 Games was to have something to take my mind off my arm and the jetlag, so, when Dave Castro announced on the first morning that we'd be flying out to his CrossFit ranch in Aromas, California for the first three workouts, all thoughts of arms, shoulders, jetlag and visas (bloody visas!) suddenly disappeared. We'd had off-site events before in the CrossFit games but this was on a different scale.

The first event was a mixed trail run, i.e. men and women running together, much like my very first CrossFit competition back in 2009. I remember lining up at the start line. The heat was intense, but not nearly as intense as the atmosphere. Everybody is so pumped at the start of the Games and the best way to start them from an entertainment point of view is definitely with a mixed event. The length of the race was only 4.3 miles/7km but the terrain was brutal. I ended up finishing third overall in the race behind Mat Fraser and Josh Bridges, but that's not the best part. About a quarter of a mile from the end I was lying fourth and the man in between me and a third-place finish was Brent Fikowski. Brent was obviously struggling a bit on the last stretch and so I took full advantage and put my foot down. Memories of letting Froning pull away in the 2014 live announcement flashed before my eyes, so now if I have the chance of beating someone, male or female, I take it. Don't feel sorry for him. He'd have done the same to me! There's actually a photograph of me passing Brent and occasionally it circulates on social media. He's never been allowed to live it down, poor Brent.

If anybody had suggested to me prior to the Games that I'd end up winning the first workout by about 50 seconds (on the female side), I'd have laughed them out of the room. Honestly! It's not that I'd lost my competitiveness or my confidence. It was that once again, as well as being grateful to be there, I was preoccupied with getting through each workout in one piece. That had been my ambition going into the Games, which made the win even sweeter. Now, where have I heard that before?

In truth, the trail run was tailor-made for me. Preparation aside, my engine was still in full working order and with a little bit of adrenalin thrown in I was always going to be in with a chance. It was workouts two to fifteen that worried me. Funnily enough, my results in the events overall were probably less of a mixed bag than they were in 2015, and in events two to five, which were a ranch deadlift ladder, ranch mini chipper, 500-metre ocean swim and Murph, I finished thirteenth, sixth, ninth and fourth.

In between events I would spend time with James and another therapist from Active Life Rx, getting my shoulder ready so my arm would work. Adrenalin is a wonderful thing. I'd get through each workout with no pain and my arm feeling under control, then as soon as the workout was done the adrenalin would switch off and we'd have to start the process again.

The closest I came to coming unstuck during the Games was during Murph, which was event number five. As you know, Murph features – among other movements – 200 press-ups, and after the first thirty or so my arm started not wanting to work. I stopped myself from panicking when this happened and instead worked out how to compensate. What's quite funny is that every time it happened I'd simply roll onto the floor so it must have looked really bizarre. I ended up having to perform a kind of weird and very wide hands-turned-in type of press-up and astonishingly it worked. In fact, I ended up finishing fourth in the event. In hindsight, I'm obviously very lucky that my arm didn't get to a state where I couldn't compete. Thank goodness for adrenalin and improvisation!

The highlight from the events, at least as far as I'm concerned, was a new one called the Climbing Snail. This one took place on the Saturday morning and when we were given the details I remember feeling my stomach lurch – again. The first part was okay, a 500-metre berm run (up and down steps around the stadium), but the two rope ascents with the rope hanging 5 feet/1.5 metres from the ground, the 40-foot/12-metre snail push and the two final rope ascents – it was also three rounds for time, by the way – weren't exactly easy on the arms. If adrenalin was going to get me through this one, I was going to need about ten gallons. The snail, which was basically a huge padded cylinder with a barrel inside, had been specially made by Rogue and each one weighed 400lb/181kg. What made it so difficult to push was that the barrel inside the cylinder was only half full of sand and with the sand never really moving very far you could never get any momentum while pushing it. It was just a constant struggle.

With it being a new event, everybody was backstage warming up, trying to replicate the snail by pushing boxes with their coaches sitting on top! Those in heat one would have to figure out the technique fast and rumours filtered back whose technique was the best. Iceland's Thuridur Helgadottir seemed to get the best handle on the snail and did so by going in low. Whatever happened, it was certainly going to be interesting.

Believe it or not, I was actually sitting in third position overall at this point and that was even after finishing thirty-third in the previous day's, guess what … strength event, the squat clean pyramid. Nobody was more surprised by this than me.

Starting the event with a 500-metre run was ideal for me as it allowed me to settle in and loosen up a bit. I think I finished the first run in second place and, when I jumped for the first rope climb, I felt great and the arm seemed fine pulling. The same with the snail; I just ran full pelt at it and didn't stop moving until I crossed the marker. I love practising new movements so that became my main focus for the event.

By the time we got to the end of the second run, which was basically a circuit of the stadium concourse, I'd taken the lead. My arm was still working as normal so James had obviously done a fantastic job. Keeping me competing must be like keeping a classic car going. You have to spend a bit more time on it than you would a new one but because it's older you appreciate the results more. I certainly did. The temperature, which was in the mid-thirties, was scorching and was making the black snails hot to touch, but I was just concentrating on keeping moving and holding onto that lead. Once I get the momentum going I find it very hard to give up and these were vital points I'd pick up.

On completing the final run, which had a very welcome decline on the final 100 metres or so, I had a healthy lead over Kristin Holte, Kari Pearce and Sara Sigmundsdottir and, with the current overall leader, Tia-Clair Toomey, being further down the field, it looked like it would be a good win for me, if I could hold onto that lead!

When I was on my final rope climbs I was starting to blow a bit but I had one thing on my mind, even when the heat started to take effect and the ropes seemed to get higher to climb: *If it's an event I can win, I have to push and get those points* – and, boy, was I pushing!

Something else that became very real again when entering the stadium was the crowd. I know I've said it before in this book but the support they give you is like having an extra limb sometimes and at the time I needed one – literally and metaphorically! The cheers from the crowd enable you to push and even though you feel you've reached your limit you find something more, something you can never find in training, and that's why I love competing so much.

The time to beat from the first heat was 13:19.56 and I managed it in 12:33.44. Not bad for an old classic. I was like a million degrees afterwards though! With Kari Pearce finishing about 40 seconds behind me and Tia Toomey back in thirteenth, I took the lead overall.

You're probably expecting this but the next few events didn't go as well, with nineteenth- and fifteenth-place finishes, which saw me ending the Saturday in fourth place behind Tia, Katrin and Sara. Starting the final day, I wasn't confident in holding onto that position as it started with a 280-foot/85-metre handstand walk, followed by an 840-foot/256-metre shuttle sprint and a 560-foot/170-metre plough drag, each portion being worth fifty points. Knowing that the handstand walk and sprint wouldn't be the best for me (I managed to come twenty-sixth and fifteenth respectively), I knew that I had to give everything I had on the plough to salvage some points.

Again, the plough was a new piece of equipment developed by Rogue and essentially it was a two-handled heavy chunk of metal we would have to drag up the field and back down again. I was slightly behind the rest of the field to the halfway point but, as the hamstrings began to set on fire and the rest of the field slowed down, I dug into the pain cave more and kept my pace. It was soon a three woman race between Katrin, Sara and myself. As I slowly passed Sara, I had Katrin in my sights and was starting to gain on her. We were sharing a lane and I was digging as far into my reserves as I could to make a final surge when she zigzagged in front of me, preventing me from passing. We both collapsed onto the finish line in agony, me a mere second after her in second place. In CrossFit you can never normally affect someone else's performance like that; it's all just about what you're physically capable of compared to the next person. I don't think Katrin was making a tactical decision to cut in front of me, as brilliant as it was; that far into a maximal effort event the brain isn't functioning like that. She was simply trying to win, just like I was!

This second place and a sixth in event fourteen meant I would go into the final workout still in fourth position overall. A great position to be in other than the fact I was now faced with another challenge – the dreaded pegboard. The pegboard already had a reputation for being one of the most difficult movements in CrossFit. The last time they used it at the Games, twenty-five of the thirty-seven athletes taking part didn't manage to complete a single climb of it!

The workout, which was called Redemption, although it should have been called Torture, was a mixture of thrusters and pegboard climbs. The weight rope double-unders in the last workout had really put my shoulder through it so I wasn't sure how it was going to respond to this challenge. I was looking forward to it like a hole in the head. With Sara Sigmundsdottir in third and a good few points ahead of me, and an event I wasn't overly confident in, I knew that realistically it meant I wasn't going to get onto the podium. The best I could do was to hold onto my position. Fourth though – I knew I'd be more than happy with that spot, so let's go fight for it!

The big story towards the end of the Games was who was going to finish first (no surprise there) and it all came down to the last event. Over the five days there'd been eleven lead changes and no fewer than five athletes had held the top spot. It just goes to show how competitive the field was. In 2015, Tia Toomey had finished second behind Katrin Davidsdottir, and as we attempted our first pegboard ascent in the final heat they commanded the same positions. Tia finished eighth in the final workout, whereas Katrin finished twelfth but, because it was so close between them overall, nobody knew who'd won. It took Dave Castro and his team what seemed like forever to do the sums but in the end Katrin was crowned the winner by just eleven points. What a finish! I felt sorry for Tia but there was no doubt she'd be back next year. In 2015 people had been saying, 'Tia who?' Now everybody knew exactly who Tia Toomey was and there was no doubt in my mind that she was a champion in waiting. I wonder what happened to her?

At the end of the CrossFit Games, most athletes will take stock and perhaps put their feet up for a few days. Unfortunately, rather than enjoying a few days in LA, I had to fly straight back to the UK – you know, that visa thing.

After the Games my training was drastically reduced yet the shoulder wasn't getting any better, so it was time to schedule an MRI scan. The consultant said there was nothing left in the front of my shoulder to help stabilise it. That was a bit of a shock. He also said that if I wished to continue with CrossFit I had no choice other than to get it fixed. That was an even bigger shock. Although

I'd had my share of injuries, this was the first time I would have to undergo surgery!

I tried to look on the bright side. An athlete I knew called Emma McQuaid had had to have shoulder surgery after the Regionals and I'd seen her lifting again in next to no time. This gave me a bit of hope so I reached out to her, and after she put me in touch with her surgeon, who was based in Ireland, we scheduled an appointment. He specialised in getting rugby players back into training within fifteen weeks and he worked closely with a physiotherapist who would devise an aggressive rehab protocol. After having a chat, he said that providing the surgery went well I could be back doing everything within that same fifteen weeks. That wasn't too bad. I ended up having surgery for a labrum and bicep tendon repair and an AC joint excision. It was obviously long overdue.

I remember posting a series of photos on Instagram telling the story of what was happening. The first one was a photo of me training with a strap on my arm, accompanied by an explanation of what had happened to it. The second was a photo of the actual surgical procedure entitled 'A little tidy up needed!' After that I posted a photo of me in my hospital bed pulling a stupid face and giving a thumbs up entitled 'Now the recovery starts'. Well, it was easier than just writing it all down. And it was more fun.

After doing as I was told and managing to be patient, I got back to full training in about fifteen weeks. I wasn't at full strength, of course, but I could perform every movement comfortably and without any serious pain. And in fact, under careful observation and guidance from the surgeon's physiotherapist Lynda Brudenell and my coach James, I was actually able to start qualifying workouts from week seven. After numerous talks with James, we'd agreed I could do the qualifiers as long as they were movements I'd been cleared to do and nothing that would put my recovery in jeopardy. Luckily, muscle-ups didn't come up as I would have been stuck then!

Incidentally, when I started my rehab, James Jowsey suggested we start working together full time again, but under one strict condition: that he did all of my programming. This was to ensure that I didn't overdo things while in rehab and, with me being, shall we say, a little bit overzealous sometimes, it seemed like a great idea. Programming for athletes is something I was doing quite a lot of at the time and I specialised in helping strength athletes develop a better engine. When it came to my own programming, I had no idea about progressive loading to rehab after surgery so I was happy to let James take the lead.

I think a lot of my injuries come from the fact that I entered the sport so late. The problem with the AC joint, for instance, according to the surgeon, had happened because of a fall and the only thing I could put it down to was mountain biking. Some of the falls I had competing in mountain biking were pretty bad ones so it all made sense to me. The thing is, because I wasn't lifting at the time, the problem had never come to light and, by the time it did, I was, how can I put it, already of a certain age. Then again, there are a lot of people younger than me in CrossFit who have suffered more injuries so it's not an exact science. Some of it's simply down to luck. Or should I say, bad luck.

In October, about a month after the surgery, I received an invitation to take part in the CrossFit Invitational, which usually falls towards the end of November. But instead of being invited to take part as an athlete I'd been invited to take part as a coach. In 2015 I'd received the same invitation and I had been upset that I was asked as a coach – although I still accepted, wanting to be part of the event, I did feel like it was CrossFit trying to put me out to pasture. Now, in 2016, only a month out of surgery, I was overjoyed to receive this invitation, knowing full well I wouldn't have been 100 per cent fit to participate as a competitor. I was much better put to use with my coach's cap on.

I also remembered some of the fun we'd had in 2015. As well as Katrin and Sara, I'd had Jonne Koski and Bjorgvin Karl Gudmundsson on my team and the four had worked really well together. The thing I remember most about the competition is laughing a lot. All four athletes have a really good sense of humour and, despite us finishing last out of four teams (USA, Canada, Pacific and Europe) with a woeful six points, it had been a good experience. However, I also knew the score wasn't indicative of what the team was capable of. I knew that this year we could put on a better showing.

Looking back, I think the injury I suffered in 2016 affected me a lot more than the broken foot. It probably brought home the fact that one day, hopefully in the very distant future, I wouldn't be able to compete at the highest level. Some say age is just a number and, although that's a very positive message, it's a number you have to take notice of occasionally. The only way not to be beaten by it is to align your ambitions and behaviour with your current ability. Failure to do that will normally result in a downward spiral of disappointment so it's something that has to be worked on almost constantly. Get it right and you'll be onto a good thing. Just ask Rich Froning. Since 2015 he's competed in the team division at the Games instead of as an individual and, would you believe it, he's been on the winning team four out of five times. Is he still capable of winning the CrossFit Games as an individual? Who knows? Things have changed and, most importantly, so have Rich's priorities.

From my own point of view, I knew the biggest battle I would face over the coming months of my rehabilitation would be with my own mind. It's a paradox really. You're dying to compete and your first foe is often yourself! What I had to try to accept was that I was no longer at the peak of my physical powers. My injury had made me think that maybe my body was trying to tell me it was time to stop. I had worked with James and dedicated myself to my rehab just to see if it was actually possible for me to get back to fitness. Now the challenge was to see if my body could ever be a force to be reckoned with again.

CHAPTER 24:

I WANT TO GO TO DUBAI!

By the time the 2016 Invitational took place in November, I was back to my old self again, and the team, which consisted of Katrin, Sara, Bjorgvin and Lukas Hogberg, were in fantastic form. Trying to sound like an actual coach for a moment! I had over the years completed all of my CrossFit certifications, I was a certified British Weightlifting instructor and a qualified personal trainer, so, although it was a kind of token role, I did have some qualifications for the job.

Coaching seasoned athletes for a competition like this is obviously a lot different to coaching, for instance, members of the public in a gym. The athletes, who are used to competing individually and have a very tight grip on their training schedules, need to be taught, or, in some cases just reminded, how to act and compete within a team environment. This can involve anything from reminding them to tag somebody (it's actually really easy to forget) to just communicating effectively. Some things, such as offering support to your fellow athletes, are already prerequisites within CrossFit so to be honest it's not the most difficult job in the world.

In all, I only had two days with the team (the other three teams had at least a day more) and when it came to choosing the training I concentrated primarily on synchronisation. When synchronising anything as a team you're forced to concentrate on each other and communicate, which promotes teamwork. Because three of the athletes had competed as a team last year, we already had a head start in that department so, basically, once we'd brought Lukas up to speed, the two days were like a refresher course.

The competition took place in Ontario, Canada, and just like every year the crowd was big and very loud. In all, there were seven events and, to demonstrate just how close the competition was, when we got to the final one there was just one point separating the first and third teams. We were first, the USA second and Pacific were third. The highlight for me so far had been watching Katrin go first in the handstand walk relay. I swear that girl can walk faster on her hands than some people can walk on their feet. She was pushed all the way by Brooke Wells from the USA but just managed to pinch it.

The final event featured a slug, which is a very similar piece of equipment to the worm we used back in 2013 when I won the competition as part of Team World. That had been as a competitor, of course, but the team to beat then was the same team to beat now – the USA. Beating them in a CrossFit competition is always going to be sweet and because I'd done it as a competitor I was now keen to do it as a coach.

I've probably made the process of setting up a team of elite athletes, doing some training and competing at a major televised competition sound quite easy. Well, for the coach I suppose it is, really. It's certainly not for the athletes though. They're the ones who have to put in the hard yards and try to win the competition.

The final event featured male and female pairs attempting three rope climbs each and thirty strict handstand push-ups. Then, as a team, thirty slug cleans, thirty jump overs and thirty slug thrusters.

The inspiration behind implements such as the slug and the worm comes from Dave Castro's time serving with the Special Operations Unit in the United States Armed Forces. The slug and worm are designed to disjoint teams apparently and bring leaders to the fore but in the practice session before the event we managed the first bit but not the second. Our one-point lead over Team USA seemed very much under threat as we went into the final event. It was clear that whichever team won this event, apart from Canada who were too far adrift, would win the competition.

After Brooke Wells had some trouble on the rope climb, Team Europe managed to beat Team USA to the slug. In fact, I believe Canada were the next team to get to it with the USA following shortly afterwards. Despite it not being as disastrous as it was in practice, our first few reps on the slug were completely out of sync and the trouble was we started too quickly. I say 'we'. I was just standing on the side lines shouting my head off, but it was technically my team. Fortunately, Dave Castro's theory that leaders come to the fore when using implements such as the slug proved correct and, after Team Europe finally slowed up a little, Katrin and then Sara took it in turns to direct the proceedings. The USA, whose only defeat in the Invitational had been to Team World in 2013, were all over the place at this point and, when my bunch moved onto the jump overs, the USA were in last place. In fact, by the time the USA started the jump overs we were over fifty reps in.

I have to say that the final ten slug thrusters performed by Team Europe were perfectly synchronised and that obviously had everything to do with their fantastic coach and the time they all spent together as a team. Well, it might have had something to do with it. It was a fantastic effort though, and when they finally crossed the line, their coach, who might not have been physically exhausted but was certainly mentally exhausted, simply exploded. Nobody had given us a chance coming into the competition so delivering such a big surprise to so many people – quite convincingly, it has to be said – was really rather nice.

I'm afraid I got a little bit too excited after the win and, after being handed a bottle of champagne, I shook it up for all I was worth and then opened it in the direction of Team USA. I'm relieved to report they took it very well. As a few of my fellow athletes will confirm, once handed a bottle of champagne, I always manage to thoroughly soak everyone around me!

Somebody asked me afterwards if I was thinking about doing this full time and it really brought the decision home. I wasn't ready to sit in the background. I wanted to be back on the competition floor!

Canada was cause for two celebrations that month, as, before the Invitational had taken place, Nicole and I had a quiet wedding in beautiful Toronto. With her being based in the USA and me in Britain, it seemed right to get married somewhere in between and so before setting off for the Invitational we decided that that's what we were going to do.

The wedding itself was a very quiet affair, which was exactly what we wanted. Nicole had two friends there and so did I. It was perfect, and afterwards we all went for cupcakes and sushi, as you do. When it came to the honeymoon, we'd actually done things back to front as before travelling to Canada we'd gone to the Cayman Islands for a couple of weeks. Not being able to see each other for such long periods had been stressful and definitely strained our relationship, but we were determined to make it work. If anything, it had to have made it stronger; if we could survive being miles apart I feel we could survive anything thrown at us. So the wedding was a commitment we made that no matter how far apart we were we would be there for each other.

The first competition I entered as a competitor after having shoulder surgery was the 2016 Dubai CrossFit Championship, which takes place every December in, surprise surprise, Dubai. To qualify you have to enter a three-week online competition similar to the Open, so I figured it would be the perfect way of easing myself back in. Yet again, because of the surgery I had no idea if I'd be able to qualify for Dubai. If it happened, great, but the idea behind entering was to test my progress and, as I just said, ease myself back in. If muscle-ups came up I'd have to drop out so it was all being done on a strict workout-by-workout basis.

I completed the first qualifying workout exactly seven weeks to the day after having surgery. From memory it comprised of a one-rep max deadlift followed by 7 minutes of burpees over the bar. Because of the injury I had to change the way I gripped the bar so as not to put too much pressure on the bicep tendon. I was confident I was strong enough, but I'd be lying if I said I wasn't a little bit nervous.

With a lot of hard work and a little bit of luck I managed to qualify for the 2016 Dubai CrossFit Championship so that was December sorted out. I couldn't wait. The past three months had been a very emotional time for me, what with the wedding, the injury and the rehabilitation. The point being that, although it had been emotional, the majority of what had taken place had actually been very positive and I was ready to channel that positivity into the competitive arena.

Some of you might be thinking, *But what about the injury? That wasn't very positive*. I'd have to disagree. Every athlete experiences injuries from time to time and the two things you have to consider, apart from the severity, are its timing and how long it will keep you out. In this instance, with James's help, I'd managed to get through the Games and had finished in fourth place. Not bad for an injury-prone 34-year-old, don't you think? Fortunately, the fixing-up bit had been able to happen afterwards and, despite it being a long rehab, I hadn't missed a single competition because of it. Most importantly, it had fixed a long-term issue that would hopefully prolong my life in competition. That's seriously positive in my book.

The Dubai Fitness Championship (DFC) is a four-day CrossFit competition and because of the sheer size of the event it always tends to attract a really good field of athletes. Since its inception in 2012 it's welcomed, among many other athletes, Annie, Sara, Jamie Greene, Alessandra Pichelli, Mat Fraser, Brent Fikowski, Bjorgvin Karl Gudmundsson, Ben Smith, Kara Saunders, Laura Horvath, Patrick Vellner and Rasmus Andersen. The list goes on and every year the event seems to go from strength to strength.

In 2016, some of the indoor workouts for the championship took place in the middle of a giant shopping centre in downtown Dubai, so in addition to having the crowd there who were seated in a grandstand you had a lot of bemused shoppers watching too. Who knows what they must have thought. A lot did stop to watch though, so, although it was a different kind of arena than we were used to, the atmosphere was still good. And we could do a bit of shopping afterwards, which was nice.

The field this year included Sara, Annie, Jen Smith, Kari Pearce, Laura Horvath and Alessandra Pichelli, so you see what I mean about the standard of athlete. As a competition it obviously doesn't have the status of the CrossFit Games but with such a strong field it provided me with the push I needed to get back to where I hoped I still belonged.

I ended up finishing the competition in second place, in between the two Dottirs – Sara and Annie. It was great to be back competing again but what this gave me above all was validation that I still had a place in CrossFit as an individual competitor. To be honest, after having surgery I had actually contemplated giving up competing for good and my mind had changed on an almost daily basis. If I was feeling good and rehab was going well I'd be okay, but if I was feeling down and rehab was hard or difficult the doubt would creep in again. The one thing I was conscious not to do, which is what drove the doubt to a certain extent, was to carry on for the sake of it and end up either making a fool of myself or injuring myself even more. I fully admit there'd been a fine line sometimes between me competing with an injury and potentially making the matter a lot worse, and it was the potential for this to go wrong that made me think about giving up. I wanted to save me – from myself.

That Christmas, Nicole and I went back to the Cayman Islands for a couple of weeks to relax and, in my case, reflect. I've had some pretty eventful years in my life but this one kind of broke the mould. People often ask me what I get up to at Christmas and the reason I think they're interested is because they probably assume that a CrossFit Christmas is quite different to a normal one. In truth, it's not actually that different really, apart from the fact that I always start the day with a big workout. After that, though, it's pretty much the same as most people's, but with perhaps a bit less alcohol. It isn't the off-season any more, so you have to remain focused.

In the year gone by, I must have experienced every emotion imaginable and, to be honest, by the time I got to the Cayman Islands I was exhausted. It's not often mental exhaustion gets the better of me but the more I reflected on the year the more I wondered how

I was still sane. The answer to that is undoubtedly Nicole and my mum, as without them it would have been unbearable at times.

I'd started off the year with the green card issue hanging over me – sorry, hanging over us – and unfortunately that was still ongoing. In between that I'd experienced the elation of getting married and the deflation of believing that my career might be over. It had been a real mishmash! The one overriding emotion I felt when reflecting on the year, apart from happiness and a certain amount of relief, was pride. I'd defied the odds on several occasions and had proved to my inner self, and to the CrossFit community, that I still had something left in the tank. That felt really, really good, and as much as I enjoyed being in the Cayman Islands with Nicole and unwinding I had one eye on 2017. If it was anywhere near as eventful as 2016, I was going to need a seatbelt.

CHAPTER 25:

I-I-I-I'VE HAD M-M-MORE THAN ENOUGH F-F-FUN FOR ONE D-DAY, THANKS

Once again, I was lucky enough to be invited to appear in a live announcement for the 2017 CrossFit Open, except this time there was a twist. Actually, there were two twists, as instead of the week one announcement taking place in the USA like it usually did, it was taking place in two different locations. The boys' head-to-head was taking place in Montreal and the girls' in Paris. Why they chose Montreal and Paris I have absolutely no idea but, with me now being based in Manchester again, Paris was a lot easier to get to and I didn't need a visa to travel there. I was up against the Norwegian athlete Kristin Holte for the head-to-head. Like me, she was an endurance athlete first and foremost (unlike me, she'd also trained as a gymnast!) and as she had been improving rapidly over the past couple of years I was looking forward to competing against her. She was young and very hungry so it was going to be fun.

The second twist I was referring to was that we weren't due to start the workout, which was taking place at Reebok CrossFit Louvre, until two o'clock in the morning. This was because it was being broadcast at 5 p.m. Pacific Standard Time, which is the time zone of California. It was the same for the boys in Canada, except they'd be starting their workout at 8 p.m. as Montreal is only three hours ahead of Los Angeles.

It didn't really register when the organisers mentioned it. I just said, yeah, that'll be awesome. Then, when I got to Paris and started looking at the clock, I began to realise what it would entail. Our days are planned out almost to the minute – eating, training, recovering and resting, etc. – and that's done for a very good reason. Start messing around with that timetable and it can have a knock-on effect. What's more, Kristin and I were a bit of a sideshow really as the boys in Montreal, Patrick Vellner and Brent Fikowski, had finished third and fourth respectively at the 2016 Games, whereas we'd finished fourth and twelfth. There's no doubt about it, they were meant as the main attraction.

Despite everybody's best efforts to create an atmosphere that made it look like it might be late afternoon, when it got to about midnight I started yawning and every few minutes I'd have to stop myself from saying, 'I should be in bed now.' The thing is, I should! At the end of the day, though, Kristin and I were in this together so, instead of curling up in a corner of the gym and going to sleep, I began soaking up the atmosphere that the vocal crowd were creating and readied myself. The workout comprised the following movements and had a time cap of 20 minutes:

10 dumbbell snatches
15 burpee box jump overs

20 dumbbell snatches

15 burpee box jump overs

30 dumbbell snatches

15 burpee box jump overs

40 dumbbell snatches

15 burpee box jump overs

50 dumbbell snatches

15 burpee box jump overs

I managed to finish about 35 seconds ahead of Kristin, and we both managed to beat the boys' times. So, despite us not getting as much sleep as them, at least we proved why girls aren't to be messed with. And why the organisers probably chose us to go on at 2 a.m. instead of worrying the boys would be asleep on the boxes!

March 14th 2017 marked a watershed in my career, as at thirty-five years of age I was old enough to compete in the Masters division at competitions. I don't want to keep focusing on my age but it felt like a big moment for me. However, I chose not to see it as an opportunity to prolong my competitive career, which is exactly what the Masters divisions do, regardless of sport. Instead, I used it as a motivation to try to remain in the individual divisions for as long as humanly possible. I certainly wasn't scared or put off by the thought of competing in the Masters. Heck no! I'm all for prolonging the competitive careers of athletes and sportspeople regardless of their ability and I knew that one day it would become my natural home. For now, though, I was happy competing as an individual and, when the 2017 Open came around, which started just over a week before my birthday, I was in a pretty good place both physically and mentally.

The second workout of the 2017 Open was to complete as many rounds and reps as possible in 12 minutes of: two rounds of a 50-feet/15-metre weighted walking lunge, sixteen toes-to-bars, eight power cleans, two rounds of 50-feet weighted walking lunge, sixteen bar muscle-ups and eight power cleans. My position after this workout was first in the world so I was managing to stave off the Masters division pretty well. Workout three, however, wasn't really in my wheelhouse and involved heavy squat snatches. I took 156th overall and, even though it would be my lowest placing in the Open, it was probably the one of which I was most proud. My goal for the workout was to get to the fifth bar which at 175lb/79kg I'd only just managed to hit for a post-surgery personal best three days earlier. I not only got to the bar but I completed four reps at it. Unfortunately, the adrenalin didn't give me the ability to complete the rounds but I gave it everything I had.

After finishing first overall in week four and twelfth in week five, I finished the 2017 CrossFit Open in twelfth position overall and I considered it a huge triumph. Remember what I said earlier about aligning your ambitions with your ability? Although there was nothing I would have liked more than to come first, realistically a top twenty finish was more than I could have asked for. The competition in general was getting fiercer by the minute, which made twelfth a huge achievement. My mentality had also shifted a bit and I was becoming a lot more philosophical about the future. Things like strength events, for instance, were becoming more and more difficult but, instead of getting upset, I simply accepted what was happening and put more effort into things I could improve on. There was no use fighting a losing battle. As a result I started enjoying myself more and any frustrations I'd felt at not being able to perform as well as I used to were gradually replaced by a sense of gratitude for what I could do and what I had.

The Meridian Regional took place in Madrid, and with no heavy barbell events I was tipped to do well. Sara Sigmundsdottir was moving regions this year, which meant there'd be a place up for grabs. The athlete being tipped to take it was Jamie Greene. Sure enough, the top five qualifiers from the Meridian Region for 2017 were Kristin Holte, me, Annie, Jamie and Thuridur Helgadottir. From my own point of view, I was happy with my performance and I'd been pipped to the post by a very determined and very in-form Kristin.

After shoulder surgery and officially turning Masters age, I'd made it back to the Games as an individual! 2017 was shaping up to be a great year so far.

I think I might already have alluded to the fact that in the weeks leading up to the Games you tend to mix in some fun stuff with your training. This year, before we left for the States, a few friends and I decided to go kayaking for a laugh and, being CrossFitters, we thought it would be fun to run around the lake first. We'd visit obstacle courses, go bouldering and take dumbbells to the docks to attempt to swim after performing thrusters! The reason for us breaking things up a bit and trying new things is that you never know what they're going to throw at you. So, if Dave Castro says, 'Okay, guys, the first workout is going to involve a 500-metre row in a kayak', at least I'll have a modicum of experience. Remember the softball throw? You've got to be a jack of all trades and a master of as many as possible.

To that end, my wife, Nicole, also decided that, because I'd had some success as a lightweight indoor rower, I should try my hand at proper rowing. You know, the kind you see at the Olympics. As much as I appreciated the gesture, I was unsure as to whether the transition from being static in a sports hall on a rowing machine to bobbing about on a lake and in a boat would be a smooth one. After all, my experiences in water haven't always been happy ones and, although I would have to categorise myself as an okay swimmer, I was still prone to the odd mishap. Or two!

The lady instructing us was of the same opinion as Nicole, in that I was obviously going to be fabulous.

'What if I'm not though?' I argued.

'You'll be fine,' said the instructor. 'Apart from the movement, there's no difference really.'

I didn't believe her.

We entered the water off a jetty with the instructor barking at us through a speaker.

'Okay then,' she shouted. 'Let's start with your arms, shall we?'

'You mean rowing with my arms?'

'That's right. Row, with your arms. Like that. That's it, Sam.'

I'd always felt very stable on a rowing machine, which I suppose helped me concentrate on rowing. Sitting on the water in a scull that's about eighteen inches wide gave me the opposite sensation and consequently I found it very hard.

'Now try using your back and your legs,' said the instructor.

'Okay,' I replied. 'I'll try my back first.'

This experiment lasted about ten seconds as the next thing I remember I was upside down in the water thinking, *What the hell happened there?* Fortunately, I was able to turn the scull around quite easily and after unceremoniously managing to haul myself back in I carried on making a fool of myself. The second time I fell in, more water got into the boat, making it harder to move and roll over. After falling in a third time, I was wet, cold and becoming increasingly miserable. I couldn't throw in the towel, though. After all, Nicole had gone to a lot of trouble. On top of which I was now drifting further from the jetty.

'Try to row back, Sam,' shouted the instructor. 'Start by only using your arms again if you have to.'

Just then the wind started to pick up and within about a minute I was at least 200 metres from the jetty and heading for the reeds on the other side. The instructor was still shouting but by now all I could hear was the sound of the water splashing against my oars as I frantically but pathetically tried moving me and my scull in the direction of the jetty.

It was no use. The wind must have been at least 25 mph and in the end I just gave in and surrendered to the elements and, ultimately, the reeds. As the cold became even colder and the water became wetter I decided to take drastic action by getting into the lake and attempted to swim, dragging the scull along with me. As I was struggling to make headway, the instructor obviously belatedly realised I had a problem, so she got into a boat and pulled up alongside me. She took hold of the scull and told me to climb onto the front. As we got closer to the jetty she said cheerily,

'Okay, Sam. Let's try again, shall we?'

By this time my hands and fingers were completely numb, as were my feet and toes. My teeth were also chattering and all I wanted to do was go and have a hot chocolate or something by a big open fire.

'Y-y-you're okay,' I stuttered. 'I-I-I-I've had m-m-more than enough f-f-fun for one d-day, thanks.'

We found out later that there are different types of sculls: a training boat for beginners, one for intermediaries and a pro boat for advanced rowers. We also discovered later that we'd been let loose on the water in a couple of pro boats. No wonder I was so useless! Nicole, on the other hand, didn't fall in once. As an ex-gymnast you can understand why, I suppose. All that balance and everything. Anyway, let's leave rowing now. Forever!

Luckily, my next adventure was to be back on dry land – though once again I was going to be in unfamiliar territory ...

CHAPTER 26:

'HEY, CROSSFITTER, GOOD LUCK!'

For the first time ever, the 2017 Games were being held outside California, in Madison, Wisconsin. I think everyone was a little bit apprehensive about this, for no other reason than we'd all got so used to competing at the StubHub Center. Also, with California being the capital of CrossFit, so to speak, it was difficult to imagine it taking place anywhere else.

Well, I don't know what Greg and his team knew that we didn't, but when I arrived in Milwaukee, 80 miles east of Madison, which is where I stayed from about three weeks prior to the Games, I completely fell in love with the place. Madison too is just gorgeous and, because it's a lot less busy and less populated than LA, that changes the entire atmosphere. Not just for the spectators, but for the athletes too. The preparation for the Games felt a lot more relaxed, which, considering we were preparing to compete in the year's main competition, was a positive change.

You could never have done this in LA, but, because Madison's so small (it has a population of about 250,000 compared to LA's 4 million), hosting the CrossFit Games was obviously a big deal and so the entire city seemed to get involved. The public didn't know your name, but if they thought you were an athlete they'd shout, 'Hey, CrossFitter, good luck!' Some bars even changed their names for the event and there were posters absolutely everywhere. It felt like a home away from home. I also remember feeling a lot less stressed than I had done in LA and that was definitely down to the location. Spectator-wise, it seemed to be more family-orientated here, and as a result there were a lot more children around. As they're ultimately the future of our sport that was obviously a positive and so all in all I was really happy with the change. There are still things I miss about LA, but things change for a reason.

One of the nicest memories I have from preparing for the Games in Madison involves a lake, a run, a swim, some coffee and a team of CrossFit athletes from Wigan. We managed to get ourselves a little house on a lake near Milwaukee and in the morning we'd get up and go for a run around it. Then, if they were in, we'd swim across the lake to where Team JST Compete were staying and we'd have coffee with them before swimming back. There was also a little gym nearby that used to open up its doors for us. As a way to begin the day it was pretty damn perfect really.

That was fun – but I was here to work, and as soon as the 2017 Games started I was fully focused on doing everything I needed to do to keep myself in contention. And it couldn't have started any better, really. After the first three workouts, in which I finished third, second and fifth, I was tied for first place with Tia-Clair Toomey. I did manage to finish first in workout number seven, the 'Assault Banger', but the rest of the events were all a bit hit and miss. The Assault Banger, by the way, consisted of 30-calorie assault bike and a 20-foot/6-metre banger. For those of you who don't know what a banger is, it's literally where you have to hit a heavy block of metal with a sledgehammer over a certain distance. Despite looking slightly ridiculous, it's incredibly hard. In fact, when we were all in a line hitting these pieces of metal with our sledgehammers, it looked like a construction site. Because of my background in the fire service I'd always wanted to attempt this at the Games but unfortunately the last time it had appeared was in 2012 when I'd been injured.

It appeared in 2017 at the end of what had been a very difficult day for me, having finished nineteenth, thirty-fourth and twenty-first in the previous three workouts. Given what I'd achieved in the first three workouts, this had been a massive disappointment so when the event was announced I wanted to redeem myself and go for the win. I came off the bike chasing Sara and Annie, so my aim changed to try to hold onto third. As my forearms were beginning to burn, I heard the announcer say that Sara and Annie looked to be slowing down. That was all the motivation I needed to dig deeper and just continuously slam the hammer into the block, over and over again. After crossing the line almost 20 seconds before Kara Saunders, who finished second, I ran to the crowd, held my sledgehammer above my head and let out a very loud '*YES!*' I was absolutely elated and, as I stood there being interviewed by Amanda Krenz, I remember thinking to myself, *This is the perfect end to the day!*

After this event I was actually back up to seventh on the leader board but the next workouts didn't really suit me. It wasn't for lack of trying, though – if only they scored you on how much effort you put in! The first was called 'Strongman's Fear' – where you had to move a 340lb/155kg yoke, two 120lb/55kg farmer's logs and drag a 310lb/140kg sled 150 feet/46 metres, performing a handstand walk when going back for the other pieces of equipment. I love strongman workouts but I'm not the biggest of athletes so moving the pieces of equipment as fast as I could was only good enough for twenty-sixth. Unfortunately, this was followed by a muscle-up and clean ladder. I can do bar muscle-ups all day but the weight for the cleans after bar five were out of my capabilities, meaning I couldn't finish the workout and took thirty-fourth.

We ended the day on a repeat of the open workout 17.5 but this time we would be completing it at men's weight and the guys would be going even heavier. I was really pleased to take fifth, and again end the day on a high!

The first workout on the last day gave me an opportunity to at least move back into the top ten and at times it was even more bonkers than the assault banger, if that were possible. It's called 'Madison Triplet' and it consists of five rounds for time of a 500-yard/450-metre run followed by seven burpee hay bale sandbag cleans using a 70lb/32kg sandbag. The bit that looked funny was the burpees over the hay bale as, because we were all scaling these huge hay bales that ran in a long continuous line across the width of the stadium, it resembled a kind of mad horse race. Instead of us going one way, though, we were obviously going back and forth, so with hay flying everywhere it really did look wonderfully chaotic.

It proved to be a tough battle between myself, Tia-Clair Toomey and Kristin Holte, although I managed to beat them both out. Afterwards Tia commented that they didn't have much hay on the farm where she grew up! I don't think Tia will have been too concerned that I beat her in that event though, as she ended up winning the Games just ahead of Kara Saunders.

As far as I was concerned, two wins out of twelve workouts wasn't a bad return and, in the end, I came ninth in the Games overall, so I was pleased to have scraped into the top ten. Above all, shock horror, I hadn't sustained a new injury. Wonders will never cease!

I was pretty happy with my placing at the 2017 Games. I had wanted to get into the top ten, so finishing ninth had achieved that. There were events where I felt like I could have or should have done better but as an athlete you always strive for perfection. Still, a top ten finish at the CrossFit Games? Come on, Briggs, that's not bad!

It's all about achieving the right mental and physical balance, which is half the battle in sport. An athlete might be the most genetically gifted human being on earth but if their mental approach isn't right they may never realise their full potential. I've seen it so many times and in so many different sports. That's why sports psychology is such a hot topic at the moment and has been for decades. It starts with the fact that all sportspeople are individuals and so no two mindsets will ever be the same. The physical process faces similar challenges, of course, as no two bodies are the same either.

Finding the right balance is not something you can perfect, by the way. To achieve that we'd have to predict the future and if I could do that I would be straight down the betting shop! What we can achieve, however, are moments of perfection where everything aligns. That's basically what we're working towards as sportspeople, either consciously or unconsciously.

In my opinion, there's no better arena to study the subject of sports psychology than CrossFit. Why? Because the variation in content and structure complements the subject itself and celebrates – and supports – the individual.

CHAPTER 27:

BIG IN BRAZIL

What I needed after the 2017 CrossFit Games was a nice trip somewhere sunny. So when CrossFit HQ called and asked if I'd like to coach Team Europe again at this year's Invitational, which just happened to be taking place in Melbourne, Australia on 5 November, I said yes. Yes please!

I'd come to terms with being a coach now and, because I knew exactly what was involved, I didn't waste any time in preparing. My team this year was going to be Annie, Sara, Jason Smith and Bjorgvin Karl Gudmundsson, and according to the journos and websites it was the most balanced team in the competition.

With everyone arriving in Melbourne on either the first or second of November, and from all four corners of the world, we were going to have precious little time to train – about two days, with any luck, so the same as last time. In order to try to counter this slightly, I set up a Facebook group with the five of us so we could at least communicate like a team before the event.

The athletes on the other teams, by the way, were, on Team Pacific: Tia-Clair Toomey, Kara Saunders, Rob Forte and James Newbury, who was also the coach; on Team USA: Tennil Reed-Beuerlein, Kari Pearce, Noah Ohlsen and Scott Panchik, with Adam Neiffer as coach; and on Team Canada: Alessandra Pichelli, Carol-Ann Reason-Thibault, Brent Fikowski and Patrick Vellner, with Camille Leblanc-Bazinet as coach.

Despite my genius idea of starting a Facebook group, our preparations were scuppered slightly when Sara fell ill during the flight over. This meant that instead of getting at least two days' training together as a team we got just one and with two new members, which wasn't ideal. In the end we didn't manage to do much synchronisation training as a foursome, as I had to step in to replace Sara during some of the training. However, they did manage to get a session on the worm in on the morning before the competition. Being positive, Sara was starting to feel better by then and she had regularly trained with Annie and Bjorgvin who were both Icelandic too, so they were already familiar with each other's technique. This meant that we just had to slot Jason in, which seemed easy to do.

The competition took place at the famous Margaret Court Arena, which just goes to show how big CrossFit was becoming in the country. Yet again, the crowds were fantastic and as we waited to be introduced to them all you could hear was them shouting, 'Aussie! Aussie! Aussie!' They obviously had the reigning women's champion on their Pacific team and when Tia was introduced the volume went up about ten notches.

Because we'd won the year before, the big question was: could we do it again? We were the favourites – along with the Aussies, who were on home turf – and even though we'd not had the preparation I'd have liked, I still felt we had the capabilities to retain the title. Unfortunately, it wasn't to be our night and, despite the efforts of the team, the lack of training time, Sara's illness and some pretty wretched jet lag meant we took last. But we mustn't dwell on the placing as everyone involved had a blast and I had two weeks travelling in Australia to look forward to!

I had qualified for DFC again so the next few weeks in Melbourne, Sydney and Brisbane were more like a box tour as opposed to a relaxing holiday. But it was definitely nice to be training in the warm weather preparing to compete, rather than freezing cold Manchester!

In December, I flew back to Dubai for the DFC. From a performance point of view it didn't quite go as I'd hoped and after finishing fourth I was reminded that, regardless of how philosophical or accepting I was becoming, at the end of the day I would always have a competitive streak. I missed the podium by about two points and it was a bittersweet experience. I had some really good events but there were a few workouts I felt I hadn't performed to the best of my abilities and that most likely cost me the podium.

I absolutely love competing in Dubai, and watching the competition grow over the years has been a pleasure. In 2018, it was announced as being the first ever CrossFit Sanctional, which not only gave the competition gravitas but meant that whoever won would be the first athlete to qualify for the Games. The prize money too is pretty big compared to most competitions so it's now become an even bigger attraction for athletes. In terms of where I like competing, Dubai is among the top, as is Australia. The people are absolutely crazy in Australia and, my word, do they love their sport. There's a real energy there and, if invitations ever arise to compete, I'll always try to say yes. I'd definitely double-check before doing seminars there again though! You probably think I just enjoy competing in warm countries, but I also had a blast in rainy Ireland! Despite the freezing cold, people came out in the thousands to watch and they're just so incredibly enthusiastic there and that genuinely lifts you up. Especially when you're struggling, it's the crowd that gets you through.

While we're on the subject of crowds, in February 2018 the powers that be at CrossFit HQ announced that this year's first live Open announcement would take place in Sao Paulo, Brazil. CrossFit is becoming very popular in South America so what better way to give it a boost than to get two athletes over there for a live announcement. They were also going to be holding a Regional there for the first time in May, so it was going to be interesting to see what all the fuss was about.

CrossFit's growth in South America brought to mind what it had been like when I started participating. The first box (CrossFit gym) in the UK had only been open for two years and nobody outside the community had really heard of it. Things were a lot more advanced in America, of course, but when I first qualified for the Games in 2010 that was the first year it had taken place in an arena as opposed to on a ranch, so the growth was happening on both ends of the scale. That's definitely one of the things I'm most grateful for: being there at the infancy of CrossFit. I feel very much a part of the sport and that's partly the reason.

In a bid to make the live announcement even more exciting for the Brazilian fans (what could be more exciting than watching me and Kristin Holte go head-to-head?), they decided to have two non-competitive CrossFitters compete alongside us, then after that the Brazilian athletes would be going head-to-head. When the event went on sale, it sold out in a matter of minutes. What surprised me most when I arrived in Sao Paulo was just how involved the people were. It was like being in LA. With the sport being quite new to the country I suppose I hadn't been expecting them to know much about us athletes, but, boy, was I wrong. Everybody I met was so enthusiastic and wanted to know everything I could possibly tell them. I've never considered myself to be a celebrity but from time to time I suppose I'm made to feel like one when people ask for autographs and selfies. In Brazil, it was like that all the time and that's pretty crazy to experience. When people saw me they'd smile and start talking about how much they were looking forward to seeing the Engine so it made me feel very welcome.

When we arrived at the arena a day or two later, the place was full to bursting with CrossFitters. There must have been four or five thousand and every announcement made over the speakers was met with a wall of noise. From a participation point of view, Brazil is up there with the most active CrossFit countries in the world. In terms of affiliates, Brazil is the second biggest country outside America and in 2018 over 19,000 Brazilian participants entered the Open. They've also had Teen and Masters athletes and under the new rules have a Games athlete representing Brazil in Madison, so it's only a matter of time before they become a major player. In many ways they already are.

When my name was announced to the crowd, the noise they created made my hairs stand on end, and when I ran into the arena every other person seemed to be pointing a mobile phone at me. It was the same when Kristin entered the arena after me and I think it took us both very much by surprise. At some point during the proceedings, one of the commentators mentioned the fact that I'd won ten Open workouts so far – wow, I hadn't realised it had been that many. Could I win another?

I ended up winning not only the head-to-head against Kristin, which was as many rounds as possible of eight toes-to-bars, ten dumbbell hang clean and jerks and a 14-calorie row in 20 minutes, but also the workout overall, which made it Open win number eleven. Brazil had certainly left its mark on me and I couldn't wait to go back.

On returning to the UK, I was feeling really positive, although the rest of the Open didn't play to my strengths. There was a max clean somewhere along the way and, although I managed a post-surgery personal best, it was only good enough for 757th in the world. I ended the Open overall in twenty-ninth position. As a competitor you always strive to do better, but it was enough to tie me in first with Emma McQuaid in Europe Central, qualifying me for the Regionals, and it was definitely something to build on at the Games. But obviously first I had the Regionals to take care of.

Little did I know I was about to be on the receiving end of another twist of fate that would place my progress to the Games in jeopardy ...

CHAPTER 28:

BEING GIVEN THE ELBOW

About two weeks before the 2018 Regionals began, I started getting a twinge in my elbow. For years I've struggled with my right elbow but it had never felt like this. I got through training, then as I was getting a massage from Charris, our in-house therapist, it started to become really painful and it didn't feel right. He said he'd just concentrate on my legs instead, so I pushed myself up off the bed and something just went. As I lay back on the bed, the pain was just getting worse and worse. It was on a completely different level to anything I'd experienced previously and it literally took my breath away.

We decided to finish the massage another day. I was doing everything I could just to try to breathe normally so I could get dressed and make my way downstairs. As I was trying to escape the gym, Mel, one of the coaches, came up and asked me if I was okay and, although it was a struggle, I just managed to tell her that I thought I'd done something to my elbow. I was literally paralysed by pain and as I spoke I could feel tears welling up in my eyes. After forcing them back, I grabbed my car keys and went to leave but unfortunately somebody had blocked me in. After catching my breath for a second I went back inside to find out who it was and ask them to move and all the time I was willing the pain to subside.

Sometimes it does after a while but this time it didn't. It just carried on. It was torture.

When I finally got into my car, I pulled out onto the road and as I drove off towards home I began crying uncontrollably. It takes a lot for me to cry and normally it has to be something very sad or very painful. The funny thing is, I had no control over the crying whatsoever and as I drove along I'd stop for a few minutes and then start again without notice. All the time my elbow felt like somebody was crushing it with a white-hot piece of metal. I couldn't take it much longer.

When I finally pulled up outside my apartment, there was somebody standing outside the building having a cigarette. Excruciating pain or not, there was no way in the world I was going to walk past somebody while in floods of tears, so after having a word with myself I managed to calm down enough to go in. When I got through the door I came to the conclusion that perhaps all I needed was a lie down. I tried this for about five seconds but because I was no longer moving the only thing I was conscious of was the pain, which hadn't subsided. The tears started again so I decided to call my flatmate. She'd gone out for a meal and when I eventually got hold of her she told me she'd come straight home but was half an hour away. There was no way I could wait half an hour. I also couldn't drive again so I called Fraser, one of the coaches at the gym, and he whizzed round and took me to the hospital. The first thing they did was take some x-rays and, once they'd been developed, a nurse came in looking very mournful and apologetic.

'Did you say you were supposed to be competing in a couple of weeks?' she said after sitting down next to me.

'That's right,' I replied. 'In Madrid for the Meridian Regional. It's really important.'

'I don't want to be the bearer of bad news,' said the nurse, 'but I'm afraid you have suffered multiple breaks in your elbow. You won't be able to compete. I'm really sorry.'

I was shocked. But the sheer pain I'd been in meant I knew that it was something serious, and I had already started coming to terms with the fact I might not be able to compete at the Regionals.

'I'm going to go and get the doctor and she can explain everything to you.'

When the nurse left, four words came into my head. Here we go again! Well, at least I was consistent.

When the doctor came in, she took one look at my arms and then stared at me in a very knowing but disapproving way. Because of the amount of pain I was in, I was breathing like I was in labour, and earlier the nurse had recommended I take morphine. But I was waiting on a reply from CrossFit to see if I was able to take it, so at this point I hadn't even taken a painkiller!

'Are you on any medication, Ms Briggs?' asked the doctor accusingly.

'Nope,' I replied as quick as a flash. 'None whatsoever.'

'Come along, Ms Briggs,' she continued. 'I'll ask you again. Are you on any medication?'

By this time I was fuming. I obviously knew what she was getting at and I disliked the suggestion almost as much as I disliked her manner.

'I'm a professional athlete and we're drugs-tested on a regular basis,' I snapped. 'I'm not on anything, I assure you.'

Despite me fighting my corner, the doctor wasn't done and her manner then changed from being accusatory and disapproving to just abrasive.

'Well, you've just bruised your tricep,' she went on.

'But the nurse said there were multiple breaks in my elbow?'

She now took a wholly dismissive tone with me, as if I'd been wasting her time.

'The nurse is incorrect,' said the doctor. 'The image isn't clear. You've just got bruising. So we need you to go home and rest then in a few days come back because you've obviously not been resting. We'll reassess then.'

A bruised tricep? I was in a whole world of pain for this just to be a bruise?!

'I'm not sure if you're aware,' I said, trying to be nice and calm in the hope she'd start cooperating with me, 'but this is my career we're discussing here. Do you think I should have an MRI scan?'

'That is not part of our procedure,' said the doctor.

'I realise that, which is why I'm willing to go private. Obviously if I need anything doing to the elbow the sooner I can get it sorted the sooner I can start recovery.'

'I said, that is not part of our procedure,' she repeated. 'Now go home, rest, and come back in a few days.'

There was no point trying to argue with her so I decided to quit while I was behind and make a run for it. After I was allowed to take morphine to help me sleep that night, we picked up some painkillers that had been prescribed for me, went back to the flat and I went straight to bed. In the morning I called my physio, Mark Stubbins, first thing and told him what had happened. He immediately sorted out a referral, which led to me having an MRI. After rushing back the results, the physio came to see me.

'What did that doctor say you had? A bruised tricep?'

'That's right.'

'That's about the only part of your elbow you haven't damaged!'

'I think I could have told them that. What's the real damage then?'

According to him, I'd ruptured my medial collateral ligament and had several fractures and floating bone pieces in the elbow joint. The pain I'd been feeling had been caused by all the bone pieces opening the joint up against the ulnar nerve. With everything pressing against it, it's no wonder I'd been in agony.

'It's not a bruised tricep then,' I said to my physio.

'What do you think?'

Had I not still been in a considerable amount of pain, I'd have been tempted to go round there and show the doctor what my bruised tricep looked like on the MRI, but there was no point.

While in the hospital I had already set off a chain of events, getting in touch with Emma McQuaid in Ireland again and asking her to reach out to the physiotherapist Lynda Brudenell and the surgeon Michael Eames to see if a broken elbow was something he could help with. After successful shoulder surgery with them, I had full confidence that they could get me through this injury. As soon as I got the MRI results, they were sent over to him and he told me to come straight over. He saw me the Friday morning and tried to fit me in later that day but there were no available beds so I was scheduled for the Monday morning. Luckily, I was now good friends with Emma so I could stay the week with her.

Each day the range on my elbow was getting better and on the Saturday I had roughly 80 per cent back, which gave me an idea. Because of the injury, I'd had to decline my invitation to the Regionals but the Masters qualifiers were taking place. And they were being conducted similarly to the Open – four workouts to be performed and filmed in a gym. The only twist was that they released all four workouts at once and you only had one week to complete them.

'If the range in my elbow is as good as it is today or better,' I said to Emma, 'how about I do the Masters qualifiers tomorrow?'

'Yeeeeeah,' she said. 'Why not!'

With my elbow now as good as new, or so I convinced myself, on the Sunday morning we strapped it up and made our way to the gym. Some people will be reading this thinking, *You're a nutcase, Briggs*, whereas others will be thinking, *Yeah, I'd probably do the same*. If you're a CrossFitter you'll probably be thinking the latter, and when I arrived at Emma's gym I felt like a cross between a naughty child and a very desperate but very excited athlete, which is exactly what I was. Because I had absolutely no idea how my elbow was going to behave, I decided to do the four workouts back to back. Had I lost the range in between workouts, I'd have been stuffed and I doubt the surgeon would have been too happy either. The first workout was, for time: four thrusters, one 15-foot/4.5-metre rope ascent, eight thrusters, two 15-foot rope ascents, twelve thrusters and three 15-foot rope ascents in a time of 10 minutes. I've seldom been as nervous before a workout, or as pumped. It was strange, though. All of a sudden the Masters was my friend. Or, to put it in CrossFit terms, my route as a competitor to the Games!

The first workout went fine. I was a little bit careful, as well I might be, but my elbow came out of it unscathed and I was hopeful that my time would be okay. Workout two was four rounds of twenty-five chest-to-bar pull-ups and five cleans in a time of 15 minutes. I saved this workout till last as I knew the pull-ups would flare the elbow up the most – as predicted, it was the most painful and I had to do a very weird technique for the cleans but I got through. Generally my elbow was behaving itself. Unlike me. There are quite a few people who would have gone absolutely crazy if they'd seen me doing this and that fact wasn't lost on me. As I said, I was just like a naughty child.

Fortunately, workouts three and four went exactly the same way as one and two and by the time we got back to Emma's house I felt like the cat who'd got the cream. Qualify or not, there was a good chance that I wouldn't be able to compete at the Games because of the injury but, if I was fit, at least I'd be in with a chance. Incidentally, the gym where I did the four workouts was called CrossFit Berserk. How incredibly fitting.

After I'd finished the qualifiers and my arm hadn't fallen off, I informed my coach that I'd managed to do them. Better to ask for forgiveness after the fact, I reckon, as I'm pretty sure he'd have said no!

Out of 250 participants in the 35–39 Masters qualifiers, I ended up finishing second behind the USA athlete Anna Tobias (née Tunnicliffe). Anna's about the same age as I am and has won the Masters division twice now at the Games, as well as having two top-ten finishes in the individual competition, so I was happy finishing behind her.

From the moment my elbow went, I'd been under the impression that my season was over and I'd come to terms with it. To be given a reprieve at the very last minute was beyond my wildest dreams really, so once again I was full of gratitude for what I'd won as opposed to what I'd lost. I was one lucky lady.

The operation, by the way, which had taken place in Ireland, was a success. The surgeon repaired the ligament and cleaned up the fragments, though he told me that unfortunately I still had a pretty messed-up joint in terms of the damage in there. But he'd done his job and I would potentially be able to compete as a Master. I just had to deal with a week in a cast followed by two in a fixed brace and a further two in a controlled brace. It's an injury I still deal with to this day and for as long as I carry on competing I'll have to do rehab and prehab work on it, but the fact is I'm still lifting and doing what I love.

Despite me having to pull out of the European Regionals, which were being held in Berlin, my hotel and travel had already been booked so I decided to go along as a cheerleader rather than cancel everything. There'd be no pom poms, but I have a good pair of lungs on me so it seemed like a really good idea. My friend from Ireland, Emma McQuaid, was going to be competing and after everything she'd done for me in putting me up and helping me qualify for the Masters I wanted to be there for her. She'd finished nineteenth worldwide in the Open that year and seventh in the Regionals the year before so we were hoping for great things. In the end she finished tenth, which wasn't enough to get her to the Games but it was still a massive effort. I was proud of her. She did manage to get there in 2019, by the way, and ended up finishing twenty-first so I was even more proud of her then!

I then attended the Meridian Regionals as a coach to Carmen Bosmans, who wanted to give me the job when she discovered I was injured. Her coach Elliot Simmonds was also competing and we'd been friends for a few years so I was more than happy to step in. When I arrived in Madrid, the people from CrossFit asked me if I'd be interested in doing a bit of commentating on some of the workouts and I said yes, why not? Because I'd trained with, or competed against, quite a few of the athletes, I was able to offer a few personal insights into their careers and performance and I think it worked overall. I certainly enjoyed myself. I have been asked if it's something I'd like to repeat one day and the honest answer is: only if I can't compete. Even in a brace, I was out of the commentary box between workouts, either training or chatting to people. Incidentally, the four athletes who qualified from the Meridian Regionals were Jamie Greene, Lauren Fisher, Oddrun Eik Gylfadottir and Stephanie Chung.

My brace was removed shortly after I returned from the Meridian Regionals, which gave me over two months to sort myself out for the Games. It was very different to the shoulder rehab as with that I'd been able to start moving it again pretty much straight away. I couldn't do much with it but at least I had some control. With the elbow it was obviously fixed, which meant that when the brace came off it was pretty much like starting from scratch. I knew what I had to do, though, and barring a complete disaster (like sustaining an injury at a very inopportune moment!) I was pretty sure I'd be good to go.

The only problem left now was the seemingly never-ending visa issue and after running into yet more problems I was left with a similar dilemma to the one I suffered in 2016. To cut a horrific and probably quite boring story short, I managed to get the team at the Office of Field Operations within the U.S. Customs and Border Protection Agency to help me out, which resulted in me again arriving for registration at the Games with literally a few hours to spare. I was beginning to make a habit of this! Had I not been able to go to the Games after everything I and everyone else involved had been through, I would have been broken, so I prayed that this would be the last time.

After you register at the Games, the organisers take a photo of you and this went straight onto my Instagram. The smile I'm wearing is huge but I think that was driven as much by relief as happiness. I was so, so glad to be there. Sometimes it seems crazy to me just how happy it makes me feel to be given the opportunity to be on that competition floor! Maybe it's the years you don't make it, be it through injury or not qualifying, that make every year you do seem all the more special?

I ended up winning six out of the eleven workouts, which wasn't too bad. The trouble is that I came way down the field of the ones I didn't win so when everything was added up at the end I was placed second behind – who else – Anna Tobias. Anna had actually won an Olympic gold medal for sailing several years ago so it was a privilege losing to her. The kind of athletes you get in Masters aren't simply people who are too old to mix it with the individuals. Anything but. People's priorities can change and they may no longer be able or want to dedicate the time needed to train at the individual level. Being an individual competitor at the Games is a full-time job.

The two workouts I struggled most with were a heavy snatch and a heavy jerk. That said, I did manage to match my post-surgery PB on the snatch and PB'd my post-surgery jerk, so despite them not winning me any medals they were good for where I was at with regards to my recovery.

We also had a dreaded handstand walk, this time over a giant ramp. This movement had appeared at the Regionals this year but because I was in a brace at the time I hadn't been able to try it. I kept failing in the warm-up area due to my elbow not being strong enough but I was able to find an unconventional way of turning my hand the wrong way round to push myself up the ramp instead of pulling. It seemed to work and was a huge win for me that I was able to get up and over it on the competition floor, although I probably looked strange doing it!

We had fewer events than the individuals so after competing I could go back to our apartment, get in my comfies and watch the others compete in their final events on my laptop, while relaxing. It was the best of both worlds really and, while the individual athletes were still at the stadium recovering post-workout, I was getting ready to go to bed! It was a definite change of pace but I welcomed it. I was still being pushed and the Masters workouts were no joke, so each night I was satisfied I'd worked hard. At the end of the day, though, had I been given a choice, I'd much rather have been at the stadium than drinking sleepy tea and reading myself a bedtime story. Any day of the week. But how times have changed. Thirty or forty years ago, athletes of mine and Anna's age wouldn't have been able to compete at anywhere near this level. That's as much down to CrossFit and its ethos as it is about individual fitness. In fact, the two probably drive each other.

CHAPTER 29

GETTING BACK ON TOP

Sometime after the 2018 Games had taken place, the people at CrossFit HQ announced that they would be getting rid of the Regionals. This took everybody completely by surprise and I think the initial reaction was one of sadness. We were all really upset and a lot of athletes were worried about what their season would look like.

Instead, they were going to take the winners from each country in the Open, as well as the top twenty athletes from the worldwide leader board. To fill in the gap competition-wise they had decided to start a series of sanctioned events, or Sanctionals. Although not actually run by CrossFit, these events would be approved by the organisation and if you managed to win one outright you got a ticket straight to the Games. There's a little bit more to it than that, but that's it in a nutshell. As I said earlier, the first competition to become a sanctioned event was the Dubai Fitness Championship. New competitions are being announced all the time and at the end of 2019 there were twenty-eight sanctioned events, in places ranging from China to United Arab Emirates to Norway to Egypt to Mexico! I'm not sure if many more will be added or how many will remain permanent fixtures in the season but at a guess I think we'll end up with around twenty really competitive Sanctionals.

The athletes who found this change hardest to accept were the ones who'd made it their goal each year to reach the Regionals. Not quite good enough to get to the Games, perhaps, the Regionals had always been their Holy Grail and so, when it was announced that they were going to be removed, people naturally had something to say. In fairness to the people at CrossFit HQ, they said the reason for all the change was because they wanted a bigger international representation, like in the Olympics, so one male and one female would qualify from every country in the Open. To then expand the competition further they sanctioned events that could then qualify the winner for the Games. So it just meant that people would now need to be focused on qualifying for sanctioned events instead of Regionals.

As well as people not liking change, there were question marks about how these modifications were going to pan out. Without them having happened yet, nobody could answer; everybody just had to sit back, watch and hope for the best. But it has worked: these changes have made the sport more international. The sanctioned events too have given CrossFit a much fuller calendar. Previously, you had the Open, the Regionals and the Games, so, apart from competitions that weren't officially CrossFit, that was basically the CrossFit calendar over and done with. Now you've got big events running all year round and from my point of view, as somebody who lives for competing, that's very good news. Before, if you didn't make it to the Regionals as an individual because of injury, that was it, your season was over. Or if you had a bad competition, which happens to everyone at some point, then you'd not qualify and have to wait until the following year. Now there are multiple chances and that's music to my ears. As importantly, in my experience, these events are really well organised and supported so once again everyone wins: the athletes, the fans and the organisers. And of course CrossFit wins.

A few weeks ago, I competed in the 2019 Filthy 150 over in Ireland and I cannot begin to tell you how much fun it was. In case you're wondering about the name, incidentally, it was because the original competition invited 150 people (50 athletes and 100 spectators), and the filthy part comes into it from the 'Filthy 50' workout. My friend Emma McQuaid ended up finishing third behind Sara and Kristin Holte and I finished fifth. As always in Ireland, the fans were electric and they even managed to drag themselves out of the bar area with their Guinnesses in hand to watch the outdoor events!

So all in all I'm in favour of the new Sanctionals, and I had the distinct pleasure of competing at, and winning, the first one, which was the aforementioned 2018 Dubai CrossFit Championship. What was really interesting about this competition was that whichever individuals won would be the first athletes to qualify for the 2019 CrossFit Games. As somebody who is quite competitive and likes being first, I really liked the sound of that.

The first workout took place on the beach at 8 a.m. local time just to the left of the famous Burj Al Arab Hotel. It consisted of a series of reps (21-15-9) for time of a dual KB (kettlebell) snatch followed by a dual KB front squat and then a 350-metre swim. The time cap was 15 minutes but what made this workout interesting was that the sea was incredibly choppy and we got thrown around all over the place. Workout two, 800 metres on an Assault AirRunner treadmill and another 350-metre swim with a 15-minute time cap, was just as eventful. We had to carry a lifeguard flotation aid with the strap removed, forcing us to navigate the ocean waves while trying to ensure we didn't lose it, otherwise we either had to swim back to shore to reclaim it or score a zero! Luckily, my single-arm-legs-flailing-in-the-air technique paid off and I managed to finish in second place for both workouts behind Sara Sigmundsdottir in workout number one and Harriet Roberts in workout number two. So far so good.

On day two we had an extra half an hour in bed so didn't start until 8.30 a.m. Lucky us! Workout three was a 2.5-mile/4km run with a 13lb/6kg weight vest into a 2.5-mile/4km run without the vest in a time cap of 90 minutes. The run took place in the desert so over sand and yet again I finished second, this time behind Mikaela Norman.

Day three started with a 1-rep max snatch where I managed a post-elbow surgery personal best of 167lb/76kg, but in the field of exceedingly strong females this was only good enough for twenty-seventh place. The woman to watch on that event was Sweden's Mia Akerlund, who put up a record-breaking 229lb/104kg, so that was impressive to watch, and incidentally she would have beaten some of the guys with that snatch!

The next two workouts went a lot better points-wise for me. I took a third place in 'Under Pressure'. The workout started with a yoke carry 396lb/180kg (redemption from the 'Strongman's Fear' at the Games), then fifteen parallette handstand push-ups followed by three rounds of fifteen box jump overs and ten ring muscle-ups, before carrying the yoke 65 feet/20 metres to the finish.

Then, to finish the day, we were introduced to 'Acid Bath'! What seems so simple on paper turned out to be one of the most painful workouts I've ever completed, and I think if you ask any athlete from Dubai that year they'd agree!

'Acid Bath' was simply 500 metres on a SkiERG (indoor skiing machine), then a 500-metre row, then 1,000 metres on a BikeERG.

The acid they're referring to is the accumulation of lactic acid in the muscles, as this workout was to be an all-out sprint. Weight can play a slight advantage on the ergs so I knew the place I could make up some ground would be on the bike; I would just have to make sure to not get too far behind off the ski and the rower, then give everything I had on the bike. I was prepared to go deep into the dark place – what I didn't know at the time was just how deep it was possible to go.

I got onto the bike in about fifth or sixth place and just buckled down and drove my legs as fast as they could go. I could see on the monitor that I was catching people and slowly overtaking them. The pain was becoming unreal though, as my legs and lungs began to burn like nothing I'd ever felt before. I was now in third ... *Come on, legs, I can go faster, I know I can.* Right then my vision became blurry and blackness started closing in. I let out an audible scream, at which point my vision started to return, but as soon as I stopped the blackness came back. There was only one thing for it: I would have to keep screaming. My poor judge didn't have a clue what was happening, and kept trying to reassure me that I was almost done.

I literally fell over the finish line at 5:33 in second place and I couldn't move until they were dragging us off the floor to start the men's heat. Watching videos back of the event is hilarious as all the athletes scramble off the bikes and attempt to run Bambi-legged to the finish. Saying that, the female winner, Laura Horvath, who finished a whole 10 seconds before me, casually strolled across – I don't even think she broke a sweat! Baffling!

I went to bed that night totally spent, but sitting in first place I was excited to start the final day! Unfortunately, I didn't stay in bed long. I'd come down with food poisoning. It started at about

10 p.m. and every hour, almost on the hour, I had to go to the loo quite urgently with violent projectile vomiting and the rest. What was nice about DCC this year was Nicole was also competing. After two major back surgeries she was back on the competition floor as part of team Central Beasts (who qualified for the Games out of a later Sanctional). So it was great to be both fit and healthy, competing together for the first time since 2015. What wasn't so nice was for her to be kept up all night by me making the sound of a dying whale.

Luckily for me, the next day started late so once the vomiting subsided I managed a couple of hours' sleep and Nicole got me some carb drinks and two boxes of Ritz crackers. I remember sitting in the athletes' briefing and I was still clutching a carb drink and a box of crackers. Had it happened the day before, I dare say it would have made more of a difference but with just a day to go I was sure I was able to get through it.

The first event wasn't the best way to start with nine rope climbs, a 40-metre handstand walk, six rope climbs, another 40-metre handstand walk, three rope climbs and a final 40-metre handstand walk. As you'll remember, handstand walking hasn't always been good to me, now try going upside down after you've spent all night with your head down the toilet! Luckily, it didn't cause too much damage as I took thirteenth and was able to eat some toast afterwards.

Now with the fuel from the toast and a can of NOCCO (a high-caffeine sports drink) inside me, I was ready to take on the world! The next event was a pyramid sprint chipper and incidentally was the first event I won. It comprised of a 65-foot/20-metre sandbag carry, ten burpee box jump overs, a 20-calorie assault bike ride, then another 65-foot/20-metre sandbag carry and ten burpee box jump overs. The time cap was just 3 minutes and when I got off the bike I was already at least two reps behind Jamie Greene and in fifth place. I remember thinking I've either gone too slow or Jamie has just made a big mistake. As she is one of the smaller athletes, you don't expect to see her get off the bike before athletes like Sara, for example. Despite me not being a natural at sprint events, the higher the expected pain threshold the better I seem to do, and as everyone started to slow during the burpees I made my move and managed the win. Just like that I was feeling great again. I think I was five points behind Jamie at that point so this gave me back the lead.

I went into the final two workouts still holding a slender lead. Jamie and Sara were the athletes closest to me and they too were obviously excited about the prospect of being the first athlete to qualify for the 2019 Games. Having your Games spot secured this early in the season would be a dream come true for any of us.

Taking a twentieth in event nine, the lift-off, meant I went into the final workout with only a one-point lead over Jamie, six over Karin Frey and seven over Sara. So basically whoever won the final event would be punching their ticket to the CrossFit Games and becoming the first ever Sanctional winner. Wow, this final would be epic! And just to add some more drama to the occasion, just before the final began it was announced that the prize money for winning event ten was increased from $3,000 to $30,000!

The final workout consisted of four rounds of six bar muscle-ups and three devils press (a combination of a dumbbell burpee and a double dumbbell snatch), into three rounds of fifteen toes-to-bar and sixty double-unders, into two rounds of thirty wall balls and five cleans finally into a 65-foot/20-metre single arm overhead lunge. They really wanted us to earn our money! By about halfway, Karin had started to fall back so it was down to just the three of us now. I had the lead but again it was slender so I had to make it count.

A commentator once said, when watching me compete, that when I smell blood I can dictate the pace and this was actually a case in point. You see, instead of chasing me, I think Jamie was trying to stay ahead of Sara who was chasing her, so this was my opportunity to open up a lead. By the time I got to the walking lunge I knew that I had it in the bag and, sure enough, as I was approaching the finish Jamie was just starting. As I stepped over the line, the commentator shouted, 'Sam Briggs, welcome back to the CrossFit Games!'

The first two people to run over and congratulate me were Jamie and Sara and, although they must have been disappointed, they seemed genuinely pleased for me. I've trained with both athletes a lot and consider them both friends so to be sharing a podium with them was very special. One of the reasons I'd entered this competition was to try to win some money to enter other competitions with a view to getting to the Games. To be honest, I never thought for a moment that I'd actually win. I obviously hoped I would but the reality was I'd just come back from injury. And I was at least ten years older than the majority of the chasing pack. Sorry, did I mention age again?

I stated earlier that, instead of concentrating on, and worrying about, strength events, I'd been shifting my attention to things I could actually improve on. One of these was swimming. All that extra emphasis and work definitely made a difference in Dubai. In fact, it was probably worth a couple of places in each of the relevant events. There were a couple of other things I'd worked on that needed improving and cumulatively they were probably the difference between me winning the competition and losing it.

I don't tend to watch myself on TV or on YouTube very often but after watching the interview with me after winning the Dubai Championship I can see I'm a different person somehow. My smile is absolutely massive and, as well as jumping about a bit while the interviewer's asking the questions, I talk at a really fast pace. Nope, that wasn't the sixteen or so energy drinks I'd devoured since the night before. It was the fact that I'd just won! Given everything that had gone on in the months leading up to this competition, I'd actually have to put it a close second behind winning the CrossFit Games. Seriously. Nobody had given me a chance going into the competition and everybody had been tipping either Jamie or Sara to win. On the face of it that was obviously understandable – I would have picked them to win too – which made the win even sweeter. I'd proved everybody wrong, even myself. To be the first ever female athlete to win a Sanctional event and to know I'd qualified for the 2019 CrossFit Games was just perfect.

CHAPTER 30:

NOT MAKING THE CUT

The enormity of winning the 2018 Dubai CrossFit Championship took a number of days to sink in. I'd been planning to take part in three or four competitions in 2019, and now that wasn't going to be necessary. In fact, one of the first things that dawned on me the following morning was that I could treat myself to an off-season! In truth, the effort of competing had actually taken quite a bit out of me, so being able to look after myself over the winter and not having to worry about qualifying for the Games was a pleasing prospect. I'd already signed up and bought plane tickets for the Australian CrossFit Championship in January. This was another Sanctional and was meant to have provided me with chance number two, should I have needed it. I'd actually been treating that competition as my big chance to qualify as I'd have been further along the rehab road. Given how much I love competing in Australia, and how fab the weather is, I was still looking forward to going. In fact, without the question of qualification hanging over me, I could almost treat it as a holiday. Almost.

I flew out to Brisbane on 1 January 2019 and with the competition not starting until the 24th I had plenty of time to acclimatise. As the majority of the athletes were Australian, there wasn't a live worldwide streaming and they wanted people to come and watch the action live. From a fan's point of view, this made being there all the more important. As a consequence, and because Australians just love watching CrossFit, the venue was packed with people.

Because every Sanctional is organised by a different team, they all have a distinct vibe and that's going to make things really interesting. With the Regionals everybody had to perform the same workouts, whereas with the Sanctionals you obviously get a variety of workouts. In Australia and Dubai, for instance, you might get more water-based events, so if that's your bag you can plan your season accordingly. At the Regionals we never saw an open water swim. It just wasn't possible. It's not an exact science, of course, but having that freedom to be inventive definitely opens things up a bit and makes each competition unique. Because of this uniqueness it's possible that each Sanctional will produce a winner with slightly different strengths so when you put them all together at the Games it'll make for an exciting show.

The first workout in Australia also took place on a beach and the setting was every bit as impressive as it had been in Dubai. I absolutely love the Gold Coast and if it wasn't twenty-four hours away from the UK I'd quite happily spend more time there.

The workout featured three rounds of 250-metre swim, thirty burpees and thirty single arm thrusters with a 45-minute time cap and I managed to complete it in 25:54. Unfortunately, that was the only workout we did on the beach and every one after that took place indoors. The athlete who pushed me the most throughout the competition was a 21-year-old Australian called Madeline Sturt. Despite her age, she'd been competing in the Open since 2012 and in the Regionals since 2014. In the 2015 Pacific Regional she finished fifth and in her debut year at the Games a year later she finished thirty-ninth. Apparently, because she was so young, people often thought Madeline was in the teen division and in 2017 somebody tried to kick her out of the warm-up area!

Despite Madeline pushing me, by the end of the second day I'd managed to win all five workouts so, together with the location and the people, I was a pretty happy bunny. Winning the first Sanctional ever had been pretty special but winning the second? At the time I didn't even want to think about it. It was just too much. Things became a little bit tighter in the final two days and my final tally after all eleven workouts was eight wins, a fifth, an eighth and a second. This gave me a final total of 1046 points to Madeline's very impressive 919. Because I'd won the first Sanctional competition, the invitation to the CrossFit Games went to Madeline and as you can imagine there were at least two very happy people on that podium. Madeline's a big talent so keep an eye out for her.

I arrived back from Australia about a month before the 2019 Open. My goal for the Open was to finish inside the top twenty, as the top twenty receive invitations to the Games. Would you believe it, I ended up finishing twentieth in the world and first in the UK, meaning that by the end of March I'd qualified no fewer than four times for the 2019 CrossFit Games. Becoming the UK national champion was a big thrill as, despite finishing first in the UK previously in the Open, it had never really meant anything before. Fittest on earth is obviously the pinnacle but fittest in the UK isn't bad either. Subsequently, this was the title that earned me my place in the Games so the place I'd earned from my win in Dubai ended up being passed down. The team at CrossFit HQ must have had their work cut out for them figuring out who qualified from where after the Open – glad I just had to do the fitness side of things!

Next stop on my post-injury comeback tour was Iceland for the 2019 Reykjavik CrossFit Championship, another Sanctional. This event hadn't been on my list until the Monday before it took place and the reason I was invited was because a member of Team JST Compete, who were due to participate over there, unfortunately injured her wrist and I was asked to take her place. JST Compete were the first gym in the UK to qualify a team into the CrossFit Games and in 2017 they finished a very respectable fifteenth. Being a self-proclaimed and sometimes frustrated team player, I was happy to help, and on the Tuesday I went to train with them for a couple of days. My three teammates, by the way, were Steve Fawcett, Jayne Eadie and Jak Cornthwaite. Training went very well and on the Thursday we all flew out to Reykjavik. Incidentally, there was never any intention of me competing with the team should they qualify for the Games. I was merely there to help them do so.

The competition took place on the Friday, Saturday and Sunday, and on all three days it was a fight between us and a team from the USA called Invictus Boston. At least two of the Invictus team had competed at the Games as individuals so we knew it was going to be tough. We ended up winning the competition on the last event and by a hair's breadth. Despite it being academic, that was qualification number five for me. Five! There was actually talk of me making it six as somebody had suggested I do the workouts for the Masters qualifiers. This would have completed the set as I'd have qualified as an individual, a Master and as part of a team, but unfortunately the workouts coincided with Reykjavik, so it was a no go. Maybe one day. Or maybe not!

The only downside to me competing in Reykjavik was that I hurt my wrist in training and it got progressively worse during the course of the competition. The injury I sustained was an inflamed tendon, which had caused a ganglion cyst to form and, although most of the time it wasn't that painful, it restricted my extension quite a bit. After I saw a surgeon, it was decided I could strap it up and continue with training, with the plan being to get it sorted out after the Games.

One of the other sanctioned events taking place in 2019 was the Rogue Invitational. Rogue are one of CrossFit's official partners (they're also one of my official sponsors) and the competition was taking place at Rogue's headquarters in the town of Columbus, Ohio. What made this competition different was the field, as it featured the top ten male and female athletes from the 2018 Games.

Running alongside the Invitational was a Legends event they'd devised that would feature a host of past champions, and when the organisers got in touch they invited me to compete in both events. Given the quality of the field, I was obviously tempted to go for the Invitational, but after thinking it through and talking to my coach I decided to just go for the Legends event instead. My wrist was still a bit delicate and with the Games coming up in just a few months I'd soon have a chance to compete against the very best again. It was a close call, though.

Apart from Rebecca Voigt, I was the only Rogue Legend on the female side who hadn't actually retired as an individual so that obviously gave me a bit of a head start. My fellow Legends were Kristan Clever, Julie Foucher, Christy Phillips, Tanya Wagner, Rebecca Voigt and Annie Sakamoto. We must have had about a thousand CrossFit Games appearances between us and a lot of podiums so there was definitely a bit of experience there. I have to say that being called a Legend is miles better than being referred to as a 'seasoned athlete'. That seems to be the stock-in-trade description for me these days and I'm probably going to have to get used to it. I thought seasoned meant being covered in salt and pepper?!

I had a great weekend and, although the Legends event was more of a showcase than a competition, the workouts were a great test. Annie Sakamoto made a really good point when being interviewed afterwards by Amanda Krenz. When asked why the Rogue Legends event was good for the CrossFit community, she said that, as well as honouring people who've been doing it for a long time, it shows the potential of the sport at the other end of the age scale, in that, regardless of whether you're a professional or a regular CrossFitter, you can carry on doing CrossFit forever. Good point, Annie.

If you want another example of bad luck through injury then look no further than Julie Foucher. Julie started CrossFit in 2009 while earning her undergraduate degree at university. In just one year she qualified for the 2010 CrossFit Games and was placed fifth. She went on to compete for the next four years, finishing no lower than fifth at the Games and earning a spot on Team USA at the 2012 and 2014 CrossFit Invitational. Then, during the 2015 Central Regional, her Achilles tendon ruptured and, unfortunately, that was it. The following year Julie was shifting her focus to med school and so this was to be her swansong. The saddest part is that Julie was tipped to win the Games that year so there'll always be a question of what could have been. Like me, she's always been very philosophical about what happened and claims it was a consequence of her pushing her body to the limits. She was a phenomenal athlete and I had the pleasure of competing with her on Rogue Team Black during the CrossFit Team Series. The one that got away.

The 2019 CrossFit Games, which took place on 1–4 August, had a very different feel to it and the main reason for this was the number of athletes taking part and the number of places they all hailed from. Prior to this Games, the vast majority had come from the USA. In 2019, no fewer than 114 countries were represented at the CrossFit Games so it had become a truly global competition. To celebrate this, the organisers arranged a kind of Olympic Games-style opening ceremony, complete with flag bearers and hundreds of waving athletes. Our flag bearer was Elliot Simmonds, who, as well as being the 2019 male national champion, had finished second at the Meridian Regional in 2018 and twenty-sixth at the Games. The UK sent twelve athletes in all and I must admit that, when all 489 athletes (that's everybody – teams, individuals and Masters from around the world) were lined up at one end of the stadium with the flags flying, it was quite impressive.

The similarities between the opening ceremonies of the CrossFit Games and the Olympic Games ceased the moment Dave Castro walked onto the field carrying a microphone. Evidently the unpredictable 'ready for anything' quality that has always been at the very heart of the CrossFit Games was about to resume.

'For individual event one,' said Dave, 'I'd like you athletes to turn around and face the screen.'

There was a huge replay screen at the end of the stadium behind us and when we all turned around there was a browser on the screen and somebody was logging into the CrossFit website. You don't get that at the Olympic Games! There was a page on the website announcing and explaining the workout, which was a 400-metre run, three legless rope climbs and seven snatches – four rounds for time.

After informing us that the snatches were squat, Dave said, 'Go warm up,' and that was it. The ceremonial part had lasted only until the athletes were in place. The 2019 CrossFit Games were about to begin.

I finished eighth in the first event, after which the organisers cut half the field, so in both individual categories we were left with just seventy-five athletes. I have to say I felt sorry for the athletes who were cut. Some of them had travelled thousands of miles just to compete in one workout. A brutal but deemed necessary cut!

The next workout was an 800-metre row, sixty-six KB jerks and a 132-foot/40-metre handstand walk with a 10-minute time cap. I knew this would be a serious test for the elbow, but with such big cuts being made I knew I would have to push and take risks. After the sixty-six jerks, the lock-out was already taxed but I shook my arms off and completed the first 44-foot/13-metre segment of the handstand walk. The feeling of fatigue in the arms and shoulders was getting real and the fear of failing the walk was creeping in. I pushed it aside and went for the next 44-foot walk and made it across the line. Seeing others finishing all around me I knew I would have to go for it and attempt the next segment, so shaking my arms off again I kicked up and began to walk on my hands.

The only problem was my right arm was starting to bend more and more with each step, so as I was approaching the final line I looked more like the scary girl from *The Ring* as opposed to a gymnast! One step away from the finish, my arm finally gave way, and, as the 132 feet had to be completed in 44-foot unbroken segments, I had to go back to the last line and attempt that distance again.

Now the arms and shoulders were even more fatigued and more people were crossing the finish line around me. I shut my mind off to everything going on around me and just concentrated on my breathing. I knew I would realistically only have one more attempt left in me so deep breath in and go. I managed to cross the line in 9:15, giving me a forty-ninth placing on that event and putting me just inside the top twenty. At this point they cut the field again to fifty.

The three workouts on the Friday I felt tested a good variety of domains, with a long weighted run, followed by a sprint workout with a prowler and bar muscle-ups, then a classic CrossFit girl 'Mary' (as many rounds as possible in 20 minutes of five handstand push-ups, ten alternating single-leg squats and fifteen pull-ups) rounding out the day. I yielded a fourth, a twenty-fourth and a ninth, placing me in fifteenth when they then cut down to just twenty athletes.

It didn't stop there, though, as after the first event on the Saturday we were going to be cut to just ten. In 2018, no fewer than thirty-seven athletes had competed in the final women's individual event so the fact that we were already down to just twenty, and would soon be down to ten, felt demoralising. As I was lying fifteenth after the final event on Friday, in order to make the cut I was going to need a workout that really suited me and performance that would probably rank among my best ever.

Unfortunately, I came unstuck at the very first hurdle as when they finally announced the workout they said two words I'd been dreading – sprint course. Typical! Naturally, I feared the worst. In fact, it was going to take a miracle for me to get beyond this point and the only way I could see it happening was if at least all the athletes were disqualified. Fat chance.

Before the event started, I tried to remain positive, telling myself that anything could happen. I did all my sprint drills and warm-ups. I even tried some mental imagery. I was a cheetah! I know it sounds bonkers but I was willing to try anything. I even tried some of Jen Smith's caffeine gum as I knew she was a good sprinter so if it was good enough for her surely it would help me? Instead, it made me feel sick so that was quickly spat into the rubbish! Back to the cheetah it was. I managed to conjure the image fairly well, repeating to myself, *I am a cheetah, I am the fastest and nothing can beat me!* But when it came to transmogrifying that image into the event itself I fell a bit flat. Bar one athlete who received a penalty for straying out of their lane, I was the slowest athlete out there and finished in a disastrous nineteenth. Blast, my poor cheetah was a slow-twitch cheetah!

After coming twentieth in the Open, my aim for this year had been to finish inside the top ten and the fact that I didn't make it hurt quite a bit. The saddest and most frustrating part of this is that with six workouts still to go I felt I had more to showcase and was in with a chance of climbing into that top ten. But I was lying eighteenth, and that, whether I liked it or not, was where I'd stay. (Though actually, after the Games, an athlete in the top ten was disqualified for failing drug testing, so I'd officially finished seventeenth.)

Far be it from me to pass judgement on the decisions made by Greg and his team, who've obviously done a phenomenal job in growing the CrossFit community and promoting the sport, but everyone is entitled to an opinion. I found it hard to make sense of the drastic cuts. It meant losing a lot of top athletes who still had the potential to really shake that leader board up. Athletes who'd trained all year for this opportunity, and athletes that people had travelled from afar to watch compete. But it wasn't for me to make sense of it; I'd been cut and that was the end of my Games for 2019!

After I was cut on the Saturday morning, somebody mentioned that there was a triathlon taking place the following day in the town where our pre-Games training camp had been based. After ringing the organisers, we were told that there were one or two places left so with a lorry-load of energy and competitive spirit to expend we decided to hold our own mini-Games. If I couldn't compete at the Games, then surely a big endurance event would be the next best thing? Be careful what you wish for!

It was a mile swim followed by a 39-mile/63km bike ride and a 10-mile/16km run. The swim and the bike ride were fine and I was loving being out in the sun and getting to use my fitness. Unfortunately, on the run my feet started to blister and I was in all kinds of pain. God, I was miserable, and if I hadn't still had my competitive hat on I could have easily handed the towel in. I kept thinking, *What the hell are you doing this for, Briggs?* I could have been sitting with a beer in the stadium watching everyone else struggle! Luckily I felt better after I finished and I was then satisfied that I was sufficiently tired! So I could go back to the venue and cheer Nicole on in the final team and then enjoy some time off after the Games!

CHAPTER 31:

A WEEK IN THE LIFE

After arriving back home from the 2019 Games I had to see the surgeon for my wrist check-up, and he used a phrase I hadn't really heard until now. It was his reason as to why I'd sustained the injury which was, and I quote: 'Wear and tear due to age.' Oh great! 'Well, you will insist on competing against all these youngsters,' he continued. 'Unfortunately, your joints can't take it as well as they used to.' It wasn't so much a wake-up call. More a retire-and-go-to-sleep call! He was actually only joking but there was obviously a grain or two of truth in it. Fortunately I didn't have to have surgery; instead, it was a case of a cortisol injection and I had to wear a brace for four weeks to let it rest. I'll take that over surgery any day. As the Games is the biggest competition of the season, it was the perfect time for some forced rest, but with the Open for the 2020 season starting on 10 October 2019, normal training would soon have to resume.

If I had a pound for every time I was asked about my typical week, including what I have to eat and how I train, etc., I'd be a very wealthy woman. Even though I'm optimistic in nature, the chances of this happening are probably quite slim so I thought I'd write a few words here about what I get up to when I'm not either competing or travelling.

My home, currently, is in Manchester, UK and when I'm there I spend 90 per cent of my time in the gym (surprise, surprise), which I also co-own. These days we have two sites: TRAIN Castlefield, which is the original site, and TRAIN Heald Green. I don't think it was ever our intention to expand when starting Train Manchester but we've been pulled along by the success of the sport really and we're obviously pleased by the way it's worked out.

A few years ago, Train Manchester started running a few CrossFit competitions under the name of Rainhill Trials. The first one took place in 2013 and we had about sixty people taking part. In 2019, we had 720 at just one event and it was held at Sports City in Manchester, which is a massive indoor running track. We had thousands of entrants and because it was so popular we had to choose who could take part via a ballot system. This isn't my doing, by the way. It's all down to my partners. If I'm in the country I'll always offer my support at the events but the interest is in CrossFit, not me. It's just crazy! We actually hold six events each year now – four individual and two team – and we've even been invited back to the BodyPower Expo to put on an event there in 2020. Will Daz and I be hosting? I very much doubt it. They probably still remember us!

Incidentally, almost every single name at TRAIN Manchester has a train connotation – as in a choo-choo train. TRAIN, as in TRAIN Manchester, obviously has a double meaning but when we first applied to become a CrossFit affiliate it was rejected as our affiliate name. Nobody's sure why. Instead, we chose CrossFit Black Five and that's the affiliate I compete under – Black Five was the name of a famous class of locomotive. Our members are called and compete as Iron Horses, which was the name given to trains when they started taking over the work done by horses. Lastly, the name

Rainhill Trials refers to a famous competition held in the nineteenth century by the famous George and Robert Stephenson to see who had the fastest locomotive. The categories for the event are named after the judges for the trials: Wood, Rastrick and Kennedy. Am I the first person ever to mention steam trains in a CrossFit book? I'd say definitely! I think that's enough though, don't you?

I am a creature of habit and when competing I feel it's necessary to have healthy habits to make sure I get the best out of my training. Recovery when training at the volume and intensity we do is more important than the training we put in at the gym. Because of this, I try to get at least ten hours' sleep a night, going to bed at 9 p.m. most nights, then I normally wake up naturally around 7 a.m. After having a cold shower, which always sets me up for the day (I heartily recommend it), I'll have a juice shot made of fresh ginger, turmeric, squeezed lemon, cayenne pepper and apple cider vinegar. I tend to blend it a couple of days in advance, so by the third day it packs a real punch!

Breakfast is the same every day, regardless of what I'm doing at the gym. Incidentally, my daily intake is 3,000 calories in off-season and up to 3,500 calories around Games time. This includes 375g carbs, 175g protein and 90g fat. Breakfast is a scoop of protein powder (35g), oats (80g) with hazelnut milk and one mashed banana. Once it has done its thing in the microwave, I always top it off with a nice heaped teaspoon of peanut butter. The peanut butter is meant to be 30g but it varies as I love peanut butter.

Because I have to eat quite a lot to maintain my energy levels (the recommended daily intake for an adult male is about 2,500 calories, so 1,000 less than me), people often ask if it becomes a chore. For me, not one bit. I love eating. What's more, I'm rather good at it! In the fire service, as soon as the food was ready we tended to wolf it down as we never knew when the alarm was going to go. That particular trait appears to have stayed with me and some would say that I tend to inhale food rather than eat it.

After that it's off to the gym. But which one? If it's winter I'll always go to our warmest location first, which is the one in Heald Green. If you're in the UK you'll probably know how cold it can get in the north of England so this makes perfect sense. I tend to collect training partners like some people collect pairs of shoes so there's usually somebody there who can help me out for a bit of a push if needs be, and vice versa.

The first thing I do, regardless of which gym I'm in, is an hour-long mobility session. This is basically just an elongated warm-up and, although I don't enjoy it that much, it's as essential to my day as breakfast or a good night's sleep. The reason I don't enjoy it much is simple. I want to start training! I'm not sounding very professional here, am I?

Old traditional gym sessions would be dictated by which muscle groups we're working on, but more often in CrossFit it's done by discipline. My sessions are broken down into powerlifting, Olympic lifting, gymnastics or some sort of aerobic training or interval sessions. Consequently, most of the time we'll be working the full body.

My week normally looks like this: three sessions on a Monday, Wednesday and Friday, two sessions on a Tuesday and Saturday, then Thursday and Sunday are active recovery days. My first session on those three-a-day days is normally Olympic lifting, which takes the most concentration so I like to get it out of the way first. After taking on some energy in the form of a protein bar, chia seed pudding or a banana – and some water of course, which I sip constantly throughout the day, there'll be some sort of metcon (metabolic conditioning) or some core work.

I'll then drive to our original location in Castlefield, which is also known as the ice box. Despite it being constantly chilly, it's still my favourite gym as we put a lot of blood, sweat and tears into getting the place to look like a CrossFit gym and it definitely has a true CrossFit feel to it. That's where I'll do the remainder of my training, but before that, it's lunch. Yay, more food! The next session would be squats or deadlifts followed by accessories. To finish the day there could be intervals on a cardio machine, gymnastics or if we're getting near competition time another metcon. In the off-season I won't typically do many metcons but as we approach competition season we'll increase the number and intensity of workouts.

Because I spend so long in the gym, the last thing I want to do when I get home is to cook or prepare meals. Fortunately, I work with a meal prep company who make my lunch and evening meals for me. I have experimented over the years with my diet and I have found that having a more plant-based diet through the day helps with digestion, meaning I can get back to training a lot quicker. So for my lunch it would normally be a vegan meal, then for dinner I'll have fish, chicken or occasionally beef.

If it's a Friday I'll usually have a smile on my face as that's massage day. It's normally just a general sports massage and helps me keep on top of any niggles. I'll also see my physio on Tuesday and Thursday. Since my surgery on my elbow I have to have regular maintenance on it to try to keep full range, and he'll also look at any other area that may be bothering me to ensure things don't become a major problem.

Apart from my physio, the most important person I see is my coach, James Jowsey. He's always very busy, but because he's based in Manchester we usually manage to fit something in – we try when possible to meet on a weekly basis. After he watches how I'm moving for a bit, we'll then sit down and have a chat. This gives me an opportunity to tell him about any problems I've been having. After that he'll watch me train and if he needs to he'll adjust my programme accordingly.

The only thing I really struggle with on a daily basis is my cool down. It's the opposite to the mobility session really. With that I can't wait to start training, whereas with the cool down I can't wait to go home! I'm fine at competitions, but only because my coach is there watching me. I dare say I'm not the first person to suffer from 'cool-downitis' and I'm sure I won't be the last.

After training I'll eat again, making sure to get lots of protein in, then I'll head on home and normally after a long shower I'll slob on the sofa watching *The Simpsons* or *Family Guy* until it's time to eat again. That to me is my prize for having trained all day and, for all my claims of wanting to be busy, there is a side to me (although quite a small one) that loves being a couch potato. Then it's obviously eat again, usually protein pancakes and almond butter, then head to bed with a book.

I know some people think it's boring but one of the most positive things I do on a daily basis with regards to my health is going to bed early and getting ten hours' sleep every night. If I didn't, I wouldn't be able to train and compete like I do. It's as simple as that. Even on a weekend I still like to be in bed early; it has to be a very special occasion for me to still be up past 10 p.m.

Something else that's important to my health is going out with friends and allowing myself an occasional treat. No calorie counting, no worrying, just fun and relaxation. Because my life is so regimented – and don't get me wrong I wouldn't have it any other way – it's nice to have a break where you can switch off. This has as much to do with my mental health as it does my physical health. As tempting as it is to be saint-like all the time, you have to strike a balance. It's a good job that most of my friends are of a similar mindset and our nights out start early and we're usually home curled up on the sofa by 8 p.m.!

After a competition I always have a few days where I just ease off a bit, like, for instance, after the 2019 Australian CrossFit Championship when I went out with some friends for some good food and a couple of drinks. Then the next day we had brunch finished with some epic cookies. For a few days I allowed myself to eat what I fancied and the Aussies introduced me to Tim Tams! That was amazing!

Saturdays are usually my favourite day. I'll get to the gym a little early at about 8 a.m. to get a head start on my training so when the rest of the gang gets in I can train with them. There's normally a group of us – usually between ten and twenty people – and from 11 a.m. until around 1 or 2 p.m. we have a full-on intense training session together before going out and having something to eat. We normally get a lot done and have a good laugh while doing so. It's without doubt the highlight of my week.

Sunday is an active recovery day so I usually try not to go in the gym; instead, I'll go on a bike ride or have a swim instead. When the weather isn't too great then I'll use the bike in the gym – stupid Manchester weather! Then it's usually a day to catch up on admin, see family and do the dreaded laundry!

CHAPTER 32:

THERE'S MANY A GOOD TUNE

Back in the present day, I was now gearing up to the new 2020 season ahead of me – which actually began in 2019 this year!

The changes at the 2019 Games, although significant to the competition itself, were nothing compared to what the boys and girls at CrossFit Towers had planned in terms of changes to the 2020 Games qualification procedure. Previously, the CrossFit season had always started in March with the Open, but with the Sanctional events replacing the Regionals, the Open had to take place before the Sanctionals, if that makes sense. So, with the first Sanctional event taking place in November, the start of the 2020 season had to be brought forward by about five months to October 2019, so would effectively begin just two and a bit months after the 2019 Games. On paper, this might seem a little bit daunting but we CrossFitters were all in the same boat and we were aware we would be witnessing, and participating in, a new era for our sport; one that would hopefully help to realise its global potential and make our community bigger still.

Sure enough, because of the lack of time we all had to recover, some athletes decided not to compete in the Open and would instead try to qualify via the Sanctionals. I wasn't one of them but I completely understand why many others would make that decision.

The Games affects people in different ways (physically and mentally) and is so much more than just a four-day competition – it's the culmination of your entire year! So once that's over, and depending on how you fared and how your year's been, you'll either be fit to drop or ready to go again.

The attraction of going again and competing in the Open is that, should you qualify, you then don't have to worry about it for the rest of the season as your place is assured. That's obviously a tempting prospect. Until now we'd had to carry the possibility of not qualifying all the way to the Regionals and, although it obviously motivated you, it could play havoc with your nerves! So it was never really a question for me if I was going to compete in the Open, I signed up and thought things would just be as normal. I certainly wasn't firing on all cylinders but that's never been part of my essential criteria, usually once the first workout is under way I feel back to normal and ready to rock and roll.

The first workout was announced on 10 October 2019 and was ten rounds of eight ground-to-overheads (65lb/29kg) and ten bar-facing burpees within 15 minutes. I managed to post a time of 8:01 which put me second in the world. With all my cylinders now firing I couldn't wait for the next workout but before that was announced I received some bad news from CrossFit HQ. The adjudicators weren't happy with my video standard, which resulted in me receiving a 2:30 time penalty. This took me from second on the leader board to a lowly 292nd. Ouch! Unfortunately, they wouldn't accept a second video submission so I just had to take it on the chin.

Because of where this put me on the leader board, it was now going to be almost impossible for me to qualify for the 2020 Games via the Open. Without that motivation – and, with the disappointment of having received the penalty – I struggled finding the mental motivation but being an ever-competitive athlete I continued in the Open and managed twenty-first and eighty-ninth place respectively in the next two workouts.

By week four I had started to mentally feel a bit better and was starting to enjoy my training again. When the workout was released I was a little daunted by the weight of the clean and jerk as it was seriously near my max. But I felt up for the challenge and I cleaned the last bar like it was nothing – only to fail the jerk and feel a shooting pain in my back foot! I dropped to the floor in pain and ultimately ended up in a medical boot once again.

What's this? I hear you say. Sam Briggs, sustaining an injury? Surely not!

The entire situation was a little bit unfamiliar, really – the penalty and having the Open in October – and unfortunately my foot took the brunt. But on receiving the MRI results I was able to give a sigh of relief, as, although I'd sustained a bad sprain to the big toe joint and the top of my foot along with some severe bone bruising, nothing was broken or needed surgery. You see, there's always a bright side! I had to keep my foot and lower leg in a boot for two weeks to give the joint time to recover but that was definitely not the end of the world.

When the fifth and final workout was announced on 7 November, you'd have been forgiven for assuming that with a boot on my foot – not to mention being a good few pages down the leader board – I'd have ducked this one and stayed at home. Not a bit of it! The workout – forty muscle-ups, an 80-calorie row and 120 wall-ball shots (14lb/6kg ball to a height of 9 feet/2.7 metres) – was right up my street and, boot or no boot, I honestly thought I could win it. Most people thought I was off my box for taking part but that was normal. The prospect of finishing what had been a miserable but wholly unique competition (for me at least) with a worldwide win was tantalising to say the least and would hopefully rid me of any bad memories. Well, that was the idea.

Although I was not officially allowed to take my boot off for the workout, I used a carbon fibre insert in my training shoe in order to stop my foot from flexing. Once that was in I was good to go and I managed to do the 240 reps in 11:21, which, after everyone had been adjudicated, put me first in the world! Needless to say, I was absolutely thrilled by this and, although I still wince a bit whenever I hear the word 'penalty' mentioned, at least I was able to put the Open to bed once and for all.

The first Sanctional after the Open, and so the first opportunity to qualify for the Games, was an event in Dublin called the Filthy 150, which I mentioned earlier. I love competing in Ireland so I was really looking forward to it. Starting back in 2013, which was obviously an amazing year for CrossFit, the first Filthy 150 had just 150 people from six affiliate gyms. In 2019, however, not only had the event moved to the famous Punchestown Racecourse but the number of competitors taking part had risen to over 1,500 and the spectators numbered several times that.

I have to admit that I arrived in Dublin in November in a strange mood. I was excited to compete – or at least I thought I was – but I just couldn't find my groove and I was seriously starting to question why I was still doing this. Never one to quit, I continued with the competition and it's a good thing I did because thankfully on the third day I was back! This wasn't because I thought I could qualify for the Games, by the way. I knew I'd pretty much taken myself out of contention. No, this was all about enjoyment and appreciation. I felt like myself again and I was giving my all. I was in a beautiful setting surrounded by some wonderful people and I was doing something I loved. Simple as that.

What Dublin also gave me, apart from a great experience, was a newfound attitude of strength that would – hopefully – serve me well in Dubai the following month. I felt reinvigorated. Not just physically, but mentally too. I had clarity now, and for the first time in months. From a purely physical point of view, I should never have competed in Dublin. I should have had a rest and prepared for Dubai. The advantage it gave me mentally, however, which was just a happy accident, transcended everything.

The Dubai CrossFit Championship took place on 11–14 December 2019 and, although qualifying for the Games was in the back of my mind, I was just genuinely excited to compete. I was still on a bit of a high from Dublin and all I could think about was the competition itself. I was in a really good place mentally and just wanted to go out there and have fun.

Because of the size of the event and the prize money involved, Dubai attracted a lot of Games-level athletes like Sara Sigmundsdottir, Katrin Davidsdottir, Jamie Greene, Emily Rolfe, Alessandra Pichelli ... There were some seriously strong women in there so it's a good job I wasn't thinking too much about qualifying and was just there to do what I could. Fortunately, the quality of the field merely inspired me to perform and by the end of day one I was languishing, quite happily, at the top of the leader board.

But it wasn't just exuberance that made me perform well. I knew we had a 1-rep maximum clean and jerk event on day two so my plan was to execute workouts within my capacity to the max to make up for the events I knew I would be taking a hit on. I had to come out of the blocks and make day one work. The events on day one were as follows:

Event 1
20 sandbag cleans
150-metre swim
10 sandbag cleans
150-metre swim
5 sandbag cleans
150-metre swim
Time cap: 15 minutes

Events 2 & 3 (two-part joint event)
1km on a BikeErg static bike
1200-metre run
1km on a BikeErg
800-metre run
1km on a BikeErg
400-metre run
Score Event 2: for time
Score Event 3: slowest 1k bike
Time cap: 20 minutes

I have to admit that after day one the possibility of me qualifying for the Games started vying for my attention a bit more and reluctantly I started to take notice of who would be my biggest competition. The main threat on day two was going to be Sara, but she'd already qualified for the Games via the Open, as had the majority of the other female athletes among the top of the leader board. Realistically, the only athlete who stood between me and a place at the 2020 CrossFit Games was Emily Rolfe from Canada, so she became my focus for the remainder of the competition. Bar an outsider making a late charge, as long as I stayed in or around the top three and ahead of Emily, I knew I'd be going to Madison.

Day two had gone exactly as I thought it would and I took joint last on the clean and jerk, so I was just glad to get that event over with. Day three, as with day one, suited me down to the ground and once again I was firing on all cylinders. The first event was ten rounds of five ring muscle-ups (unbroken) and a 10-metre handstand walk (unbroken) in a time cap of 12 minutes. Everyone knows I love muscle-ups and, despite my history with handstand walks, I managed to finish fourth. The next event – seven hang snatches, seven snatches and seven squat snatches (all with 110lb/50kg weights) in 2 minutes – saw me finish in seventeenth and with Emily finishing in ninth she was able to claw a few points back. I can't remember exactly where Emily was on the leader board at this point but she was close enough for me to know she was there.

The final event of day three – a long chipper – had heavy walking lunges so I had to attack it strategically, just managing to overtake Sara on the final rope climb to win my heat. Unfortunately for me, Mikaela Norman from Sweden had posted a faster time in the previous heat! I managed to finish second though, and, when I left for the hotel that night, I did so with a thirty-four-point lead on Emily. With one day and four events to go, Emily could still beat me. In fact, she could beat me easily if I didn't perform. I just had to make sure that I did.

When we arrived for the final day of the competition I was buzzing. I'd had a great three days competing, I was having fun and was still feeling good and energised going into the last day of competition, and that's a great feeling to have. I knew I was sitting near the top of the leader board and in the golden ticket position, but qualifying was the future. This was about the here and now. I just had to give it everything I had and hopefully the rest would take care of itself.

Events one and two on the last day yielded a third and seventh position. I still didn't have it in the bag but I had a sizeable lead over Emily so I knew that, as long as there wasn't a complete disaster, I would be qualifying for the Games. My aim now was to finish on the podium as I was in fourth place going into the final two workouts. Because the final event was in two parts and they had increased the prize money of the first half to $10,000, there was the temptation to go balls-out on that part. However, if I was to avoid the aforementioned disaster and be in with a chance of climbing onto the podium, I needed to pace it and go for the overall event win. The event featured a 60-calorie ride on an Echo bike, sixty toes-to-bar (one round as fast as possible), leading into the second half of the event, which was three rounds of ten burpee box jump overs and ten thrusters (88lb/40kg), and all within 14 minutes. Bring it on!

I must have got my pacing spot on because I managed to not only win the first part of the event for the $10,000 but also muster the energy to win the final part too! The fairy-tale ending was complete. I've experienced a lot of highs in my career and, although I might be in danger of repeating myself (I think I've already claimed quite a few of these), this has to be up there with the biggest and best of them. I was beaten into third place overall by Sara Sigmundsdottir who finished first, and Karin Frey in second. I'll take that, thank you very much!

In less than three months' time I was going to be thirty-eight years old, and when I stepped onto the podium that fact wasn't lost on me. I'm not daft enough to believe that age is just a number. It isn't. Nothing lasts forever so I'm going to enjoy every moment like this I have. One day even babies like Sara, Karin and Emma McQuaid will be approaching thirty-eight. Sorry, girls. You may as well find out now!

What we have some control over is how we arrive at these great milestones (imagine what I'll be like when I get to forty?) and that, ultimately, is what keeps me going. I said before that my goals will have to change one day but, however impressive they might seem to other people, what's important is that I tackle each and every one of them in good health (barring any unfortunate injuries) and with good grace.

CHAPTER 33:

A WORLD TURNED UPSIDE-DOWN

As I write it's about eighteen months since I finished the original last chapter of this book. If I had taken bets on what would happen between September 2019 and March 2021, I would probably have given odds of about a million to one on what has actually taken place. However, at the end of the day this is a book about a CrossFit athlete from Leeds who likes to train and compete every so often, so I will try to stay on topic as much as I can.

The last time I put pen to paper, or fingers to keyboard, was December 2019. I was in Dubai and had just qualified for the 2020 CrossFit Games. The first event I entered after that was two months later in Miami. The Wodapalooza CrossFit Festival, to be exact, which took place from 20 to 23 February. I was competing as part of a team once again and was joined by Harriet Roberts, Michael Smith and Joshua Al-chamaa. Richard Froning and the Mayhem team were also competing at this event so we were obviously going to have our work cut out. We ended up finishing second, which qualified us for the Games, but as Harriet Roberts and I had already qualified as individuals we had to decline the invitation. That was always going to be the case, by the way, so nobody was disappointed. We were there to have fun and get some more competition exposure.

While the event was taking place, the world was already beginning to change because of Covid-19 but I had no idea that this would be the last time I'd compete in front of an audience for such a long period of time. If I had I might have competed as an individual. As it was, though, we made a lot of good memories so it wasn't too bad.

After Miami I flew straight to Nicole's place in Ohio. The plan was to spend a month there before returning to the UK to sort out my affairs in order to move to Ohio permanently. I wasn't getting rid of TRAIN, by the way. Or at least my interest in them. I could never do that. It was more moving out my flat. But before that could happen, Covid took a grip on the world, and my flight in to the UK in April was cancelled so I didn't make it back until November.

So, what to do in the meantime? The biggest problem Nicole and I faced was not being able to go to the gym. Or even *a* gym. Any gym would have done at the time. In the end we decided to rent a garage near our apartment and crammed it with as much equipment as we could lay our hands on. A lot of equipment was already selling out everywhere so we were literally forced to beg, borrow and steal. Actually, we didn't really steal anything but we did borrow though, and we definitely begged.

If I had not been able to train throughout lockdown I'm not sure how I'd have coped. The future of the Games that year was in doubt but, regardless of that, training is my lifeblood and not being able to do any would have been unbearable. Maintaining some kind of normality was obviously one of the main issues that everybody in lockdown had to deal with, apart from the virus itself, of course. As well as coping with the mental strain of not knowing how long we'd be locked down for.

Once the garage was full of equipment, the next problem was finding the motivation to use it. Not knowing if we had competitions to train for or anyone to train with was definitely hard at first. Fortunately, I'm a creature of habit so after really pushing myself for a few weeks I managed to make it the norm. The person, or should I say animal, who I felt most sorry for during lockdown – certainly within the radius of our apartment – was our dog. Every day he had to accompany me to the garage and watch me train for hours on end. Luckily we stayed friends as we ended each day in the dog park.

I can't go into too much detail about this for obvious reasons, nor do I wish to really, but in the spring of 2020 CrossFit's founder, Greg Glassman, made some comments on social media and on a Zoom call that were completely unacceptable and which threw the world of CrossFit into turmoil. What a year it was becoming. The only positive to all this was that the sponsors, affiliates and athletes, both professional and amateur, were united in our condemnation of Greg's comments so we knew that whatever action we took we'd be able to show a united front. Reebok were the first to act by announcing their intention to sever ties with the CrossFit brand because of Greg's comments. This was a massive game changer and, with the strength of feeling against him increasing, we had no option but to follow suit and end our association.

This obviously left us and the sport in limbo. At the end of the day, Greg owned CrossFit so if we felt we couldn't practise CrossFit what on earth were we going to do? Various tentative meetings took place about how things might pan out and for a time I genuinely didn't know what was going to happen. We weren't looking into a black hole exactly, but unless Greg agreed to sell his shares and remove himself from the CrossFit organisation completely, which we felt was what was needed in order to move forward, we had absolutely no idea what the future would look like.

Fortunately, at the eleventh hour, Greg decided to sell his shares in CrossFit to businessman Eric Roza and leave the organisation for good. Because of what had happened, though, a lot of people sat on the fence to see how it would play out, rather than immediately re-committing to CrossFit. It was a nail-biting time. Fortunately, it all turned out okay. Eric's evidently a big fan of the sport and seems to have its best interests at heart, which is all you really need from an owner or CEO. Apart from a few quid, of course! Greg must have realised that, despite his apology, if he stayed in place CrossFit could have died and so he did the right thing.

I have been asked once or twice what I think might have happened if CrossFit had ceased to exist after this situation and I'm honestly not sure. It's only ever going to be hypothetical, fortunately, but I think we'd have continued with something very similar to CrossFit but under a different name, and we'd still have crowned a champion each year. I won't deny that the thought of having to create something new and start all over again was quite scary. Anyway, thankfully it didn't come to that.

In late May, the gyms finally reopened and, with the 2020 Rogue Invitational taking place on 13 and 14 June, it happened just in the nick of time. The competition itself was the antithesis of last year's. For a start, there was obviously no crowd and the crowd at last year's Rogue had been amazing. You also weren't allowed to have anyone in the gym so the only people present apart from the athletes were an operations manager and a judge. They also couldn't shout any words of encouragement as we competed, which are as much a part of CrossFit as training itself.

All of the events were then streamed to Rogue, who then edited them and streamed them publicly. It really was weird, though.

Because it was being streamed you couldn't have any music or make any noise, apart from the noises you make naturally while competing. The grunts, etc! It obviously wasn't ideal but we just had to keep reminding ourselves that it was better than the alternative, which was nothing at all. Everyone was in the same boat, of course, so we just had to get on with it.

I finished twelfth at the 2020 Rogue, which wasn't bad, all things considered. Incidentally, the only event I won at the competition was called 'Last Man Standing'. It's an event where you have to perform an increasing number of repetitions each minute until you can't compete any more. We were doing power snatches and I ended up completing 211 reps, which was thirty-six more than my nearest competitor. Everyone was joking as if we'd done it in person I could have had the last minute off!

The one big question hanging over us all at this point was whether the 2020 CrossFit Games would still go ahead. As much as I love competing at events like Rogue, all roads lead to the CrossFit Games and the entire community was on tenterhooks. The biggest problem the athletes who'd qualified faced was to do with training. With no dates confirmed and rumours constantly circulating that the Games were going to be either postponed or cancelled, we just couldn't prepare as we normally would. Training to compete at the Games is something you do over a period of many months and the timing involved is vitally important.

After literally hundreds of rumours had done the rounds, it was eventually decided that the 2020 Games would be split into two parts – the first part featuring all thirty male and female athletes who had qualified for the Games, which would take place remotely and be streamed online, and the second part featuring the remaining five male and female athletes. For this part the athletes were going to be flown to the CrossFit ranch in California where they would compete in an in-person competition.

Having a remote CrossFit Games – at least for the first part – was going to be even stranger than having a Rogue Invitational with no crowd. That said, the news that only five athletes would be taken to the ranch was met with negativity from some quarters and there were a lot of complaints. Once again, though, what was the alternative? So many sporting events had already been cancelled throughout the world. When push came to shove, we were actually very lucky that the organisers managed to find a way to go ahead with it at all.

The competition was a bit of a mixed bag for me, or at least the first part was. I had some good events and some bad. Ultimately, though, I didn't make it to the second part of the Games, which was obviously disappointing. Not just because I wanted a chance to compete with the very best, but because it would have been amazing to go back to the ranch. Looking on the bright side, I competed in another CrossFit Games. At the time of writing, the first Open of 2021 is about two weeks away and I have every intention of trying to qualify again as an individual. In fact, I'd say that my desire to be there right at the very end is as strong, if not stronger, now as it was right at the very beginning.

The end of the Games brought to a close what had been a pretty long season. Sorry, a very long season! The first Open of 2019 had taken place in the winter and the Games had been held almost a year later. Having to remain competition fit for such a long period of time was hard work and by the time the Games had finished, or at least the first part of it, I was ready for a break.

The first thing Nicole and I did was to go and stay at a friend's lake house to chill out. I went for the odd bike ride and we dipped in and to of the lake but apart from that we did nothing. It was just pure relaxation. And no macro counting! After a few blissful days of this, I received a telephone call asking me if I would like to participate in the 2020 Spartan Games. 'Possibly,' I said to the organisers. 'It all depends on when it is.' When I asked this question I was expecting them to say early next year or something but they didn't.

'It starts in two weeks' time,' said the organisers.

'Okay then,' I said. 'I'm in.'

As eager as I am to compete, I'm under no illusions as to how much longer invitations like this will continue to come my way. So, although I could quite happily have carried on doing nothing for at least another month, I had to snatch the opportunity. Also, it was a chance to compete in an in-person tournament, which were obviously very rare at the time.

The Spartan Games is a four-day tournament featuring twelve women and twelve men from a variety of sporting backgrounds. It takes place in Vermont, and in 2020 the prize fund was a whopping $100,000. On the women's side this year we had Spartan World Champion Lindsay Webster, *Million Dollar Mile* defender Emma Chapman, 2:24:28 marathon finisher Kellyn Taylor, CrossFit athlete Kristi O'Connell, CrossFit and DEKA athlete Lauren Weeks, Spartan World Champion Nicole Mericle, adventure racer and professional acrobat Chelsey Magness, elite ultra-racer Samantha Wood, weightlifter Faith Cooke, Spartan pro and triathlete Corinna Coffin and Spartan Ultra World Champion Rea Kolbl. And on the men's side, XTERRA World Champion Josiah Middaugh, Spartan World Champion Ryan Atkins, *Million Dollar Mile* defender Max Fennell, 2008 Olympian Jarrod Shoemaker, elite Spartan pro Aaron Newell, *American Ninja Warrior's* Grant McCartney, former NFL linebacker Curt Maggitt, SERE specialist Matt Stevens, elite Spartan athlete Hunter McIntyre, ultra-marathoner Mike Wardian, elite Spartan pro Ryan Kent and CrossFit athlete Herman Demmink.

I remember asking the organisers to give me a description of the Spartan Games as I wasn't familiar with it and when they did my jaw almost hit the ground. They described it as 'twenty-four athletes from different sports all competing against each other for four days and in a variety of events'. It was manna from heaven. I was so sold! This was, in my mind, the second part of the Games. Spartan did a really good job of getting everyone Covid tested and creating a bubble so life became pretty normal for those four days.

The first day included three scored events. The 'Highland Games' was the last event of the day, which included three mini events that gave the athletes one score.

The events were the 'Spartan Cross', which was a half-mile obstacle course with eleven obstacles per lap (athletes had to do five laps), a 200-metre swim in the lake for forty-five minutes (as many laps as possible) and the aforementioned Highland Games, which included a tug of war – one on one, single elimination – 'Heavy Stones' and the 'Keiser Sled'.

Bearing in mind I only had two weeks to get competition fit (although, saying that, I'd actually had to keep myself competition fit for the best part of a year!), I actually did okay, ending the first day in fourth place. More importantly, I enjoyed every last second of it. At some point every athlete was out of their comfort zone so despite our different backgrounds we were all in the same boat. I remember watching the marathon runner Kellyn Taylor trying to lift the stones. She's tiny in stature so some of the stones were twice the size of her. Watching her get to grips with this – literally – was an inspiration and she completely defied the odds. I also remember watching the weightlifter Faith Cooke taking part in a trial run. This wasn't her best event but she was happily trotting up and down the mountain, saying, 'This is great! When am I going to get a chance to do this again?'

The next three days featured vertical climbs, mountain bike events and even wrestling! It was just awesome. Though halfway through the six-hour trial run I remember thinking to myself, 'Never again!' That was seriously hard. But I didn't mean it. I may have been out of my comfort zone in many events but I was in my element, if you see what I mean.

I finished fourth overall and the only question I had for the organisers at the end of the competition was 'Can I come back next year?' It was the first time they'd done anything that big and all in all it had been a massive success. I'm not sure if they will invite me back but, if they do, I'll snap their hands off.

After the Spartan Games I had another short rest before heading out to Germany to appear at the HYROX World Championships. HYROX is a relatively new fitness organisation and the actual competition consists of just one indoor event featuring many workouts, the culmination of which is an 8-kilometre run. During that 8km run you have to stop eight times and complete another prescribed workout. I was invited to these World Championships as a wild card – one of two CrossFit athletes – and with not a lot happening in the CrossFit world at the time (Dubai and other events had unfortunately been cancelled) it was great to be involved in another in-person competition.

The HYROX World Championships coincided with my finally getting the opportunity to sort out my permanent move to America. This had been a long time coming but I was so happy that now I could make a proper home there at last. After all the trials and tribulations Nicole and I had endured with my green card saga, it felt great to put the issue behind us once and for all.

Back in Manchester to sort my move to the US, I had what turned out to be quite a crazy idea to organise a charity event across various gyms in order to try to raise some money for Cancer Research. We decided that the event would be a 100-kilometre challenge, featuring 50 kilometres on the rower and 50 kilometres running. I haven't regretted many decisions I've made in my life but this one came very, very close. The fatigue and pain I felt were on an industrial scale but we did manage to raise over £10,000. The number of people who took part in the event was also amazing, so despite my being almost too tired to crawl on a plane to return to my new home afterwards, it was definitely worth it. Somebody asked me before I left if we were going to do the same event next year and my answer was short and to the point. 'No!' I said definitely. I literally couldn't walk for two weeks afterwards and the fact that it was my idea made it even worse. Next time I'll just hand over the money!

Because I'm older than the majority of athletes competing at my level, I'm often asked how long I can go on for. Actually, I should change that to 'always asked'. I'm not saying it gets on my nerves or anything but it would be nice if I could get through an interview without it being asked. I should take it as a compliment really, as it's proof that I'm doing something out of the ordinary. Regardless, my answer always remains the same: 'For as long as I'm able to physically and for as long as I remain competitive.' If anything, my competitive streak has grown over the years, which might cause some problems in a year or two. That's also why I find it difficult answering the other common question, which is what will I do when I stop competing. I think I'll always compete at some level. It's the reason I get out of bed.

Something that's made me think a lot less about my own future is the Covid situation and the effect that it's had on both CrossFit and the world in general. There's very little I can do about the bigger issue but seeing some light at the end of the tunnel in recent months has given us all a bit of a lift. The thing that's undoubtedly kept CrossFit together, apart from a new CEO, is our sense of community. Seeing that come to the fore during a period of such uncertainty has been heartwarming. I love competing as an individual but what makes it really special is that it's all done within a team.

As always, work hard and follow your dreams – you never know where they'll take you.

ACKNOWLEDGEMENTS

In some ways writing a book has been harder than training for the CrossFit Games. It's like being back at school! As somebody who thrives on new challenges I've given it my all and I've been helped by a great team of people. They are James Hogg, Alejandro Rueda Valido, Tim Bates at PFD, Anna Mrowiec and Michelle Warner at Ebury and last but not least, Lindsay Davies. Thanks everyone. It's been fun.

INDEX

SB indicates Sam Briggs.